Keto Diet Cookbook

*An Easy Guide To Learn
A Shortcut To Ketosis, Lose Weight,
Feel Great With The Best Ketogenic Recipes
And Keto Diet Plan*

Anne Spencer

CONTENTS

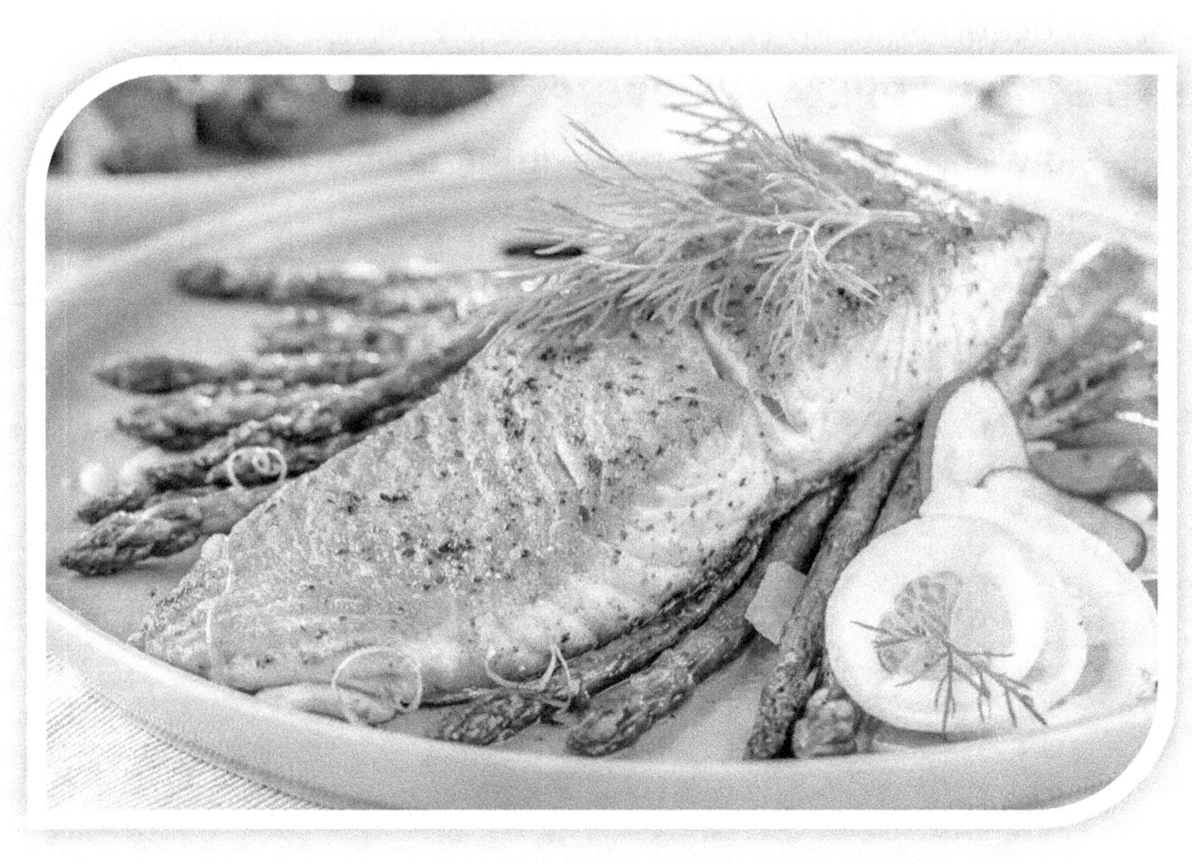

INTRODUCTION

It's widely-spread knowledge that our bodies are designed to run primarily on carbs. We use them to provide our bodies with the energy required to boost our state, exercise, or just normal body functioning. However, most people are clueless about the fact that carbs are not the only source of fuel our bodies can use. Just like they can run on carbs, our bodies can also use fat sources. When we ditch the carbs and focus on providing our bodies with more fat, we are embarking on the ketogenic train.

The ketogenic diet is not just another fad diet. It has been around since 1920 and has resulted in outstanding results and amazingly successful stories. If you are new to the keto world and have no idea what I am talking about, let me simplify this for you.

For you to truly understand what the keto diet is all about and why you should start it as soon as you can, let me first explain what happens to your body after consuming a carb-loaded meal.

Imagine you have just swallowed a giant bowl of spaghetti. Your tummy is full, your taste buds are satisfied, and your body is provided with more carbs than necessary. After consumption, your body immediately starts the process of digestion, during which your body will break down the consumed carbs into glucose, which is a source of energy your body depends on. So one might ask, "What is wrong with carbs?" For starters, there are some things: they raise the blood sugar, make your body work excessively to offset the effects of that sugar, and kindly storing it as another layer of fat, usually around the belly, but many times around the organs too. That's extremely dangerous. Sounds scary? I know.

By now, you've undoubtedly heard of the keto diet and the many people who have had success losing weight and keeping it off. But just what is a ketogenic diet, and how does it work to reach your weight loss goal.

The keto diet is a food plan that is high in fat and low in carbs. The human body uses carbohydrates as its primary fuel source; however, when fats replace carbs, the body enters a metabolic state known as "ketosis." During

ketosis, because of the lack of carbs, the body will burn stored fat as fuel, which can help you lose weight.

Not only can the keto diet promote weight loss, but it also comes with numerous health benefits:

- Management of diabetes
- Lower cholesterol
- Improved mental clarity
- Reduces the risk and symptoms of polycystic ovary syndrome (POS)
- Lower risk of some cancers
- Lower risk of cardiovascular disease

The keto diet requires a change in your wearing habits. It's easier to make these changes when you have your partner or other family members' active support. As a couple, you'll be able to encourage each other on those days that are more difficult than others for sticking to your food plan.

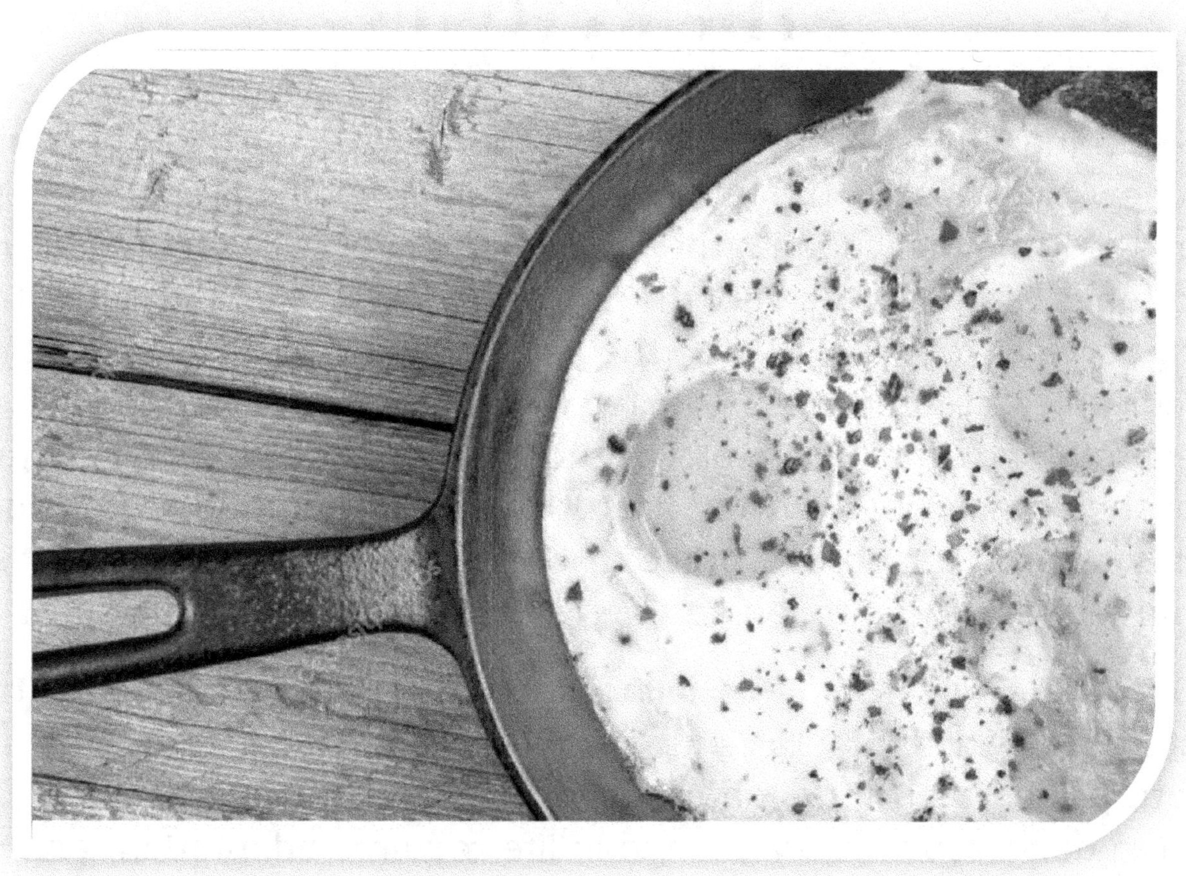

THE KETOSIS

Switching to high fat moderate protein cycle, your liver now has a new "fuel boss" - the fat. Once your liver begins preparing your body for the fuel change, the fat from the liver will start producing ketones – hence the name Ketogenic. What glucose is for the carbs, the ketones are for the fat, meaning they are the tiny molecules created once the fat is broken down to be used as energy. The switch from glucose to ketones is something that has pushed many people away from this diet. Some people consider this to be a dangerous process, but the truth is, your body will run just as efficiently on ketones as it does on glucose.

Once your body shifts to using ketones as fuel, you are in the state of ketosis. Ketosis is a metabolic process that may be interpreted as a little 'shock' to your body. However, this is far from dangerous. Every change in life requires adaptation, and so does this. This adaptation process is not set in stone, and every person goes through ketosis differently. However, for most people, it takes around 2 weeks to adapt to the new lifestyle fully.

Note! This is all biological and completely healthy. You have spent your whole life packing your body with glucose; naturally, you need time to adapt to the new dietary change.

Foods Allowed On the Keto Diet

Plan your meals and snacks around the following foods:

- Eggs
- Meats, including beef, pork, chicken, and veal
- Fish, including fish high in fat such as mackerel, trout, and salmon
- Cheeses
- Nuts and seeds, including nut and seed butter

- Cream and butter

- Avocadoes

- Healthy oils, such as olive, avocado, and coconut oils

- Low-carb vegetables, such as peppers, onions, tomatoes, and green vegetables

- Herbs and spices, including salt and pepper

To be sure you're getting enough of the right nutrients, eat a wide variety of meats, vegetables, seeds, and nuts on the allowed food list.

Foods Restricted On the Keto Diet

These are the foods that are restricted on a ketogenic food plan:

- Grains and starches, such as bread, pasta, cereal, and rice

- Carrots, potatoes, yams, sweet potatoes, and parsnips

- Beans and legumes, including chickpeas, lentils, and peas

- Fruit, except for small quantities of berries

- Sugar in any form, including foods that contain fructose

- Processed diet foods and Alcohol

- Condiments that contain sugar

- Unhealthy fats, such as processed vegetable oils and mayonnaise

- Alcohol

Getting Started with Your Keto Diet

Before starting the keto diet, take some time researching the foods on the allowed list and those restricted foods. Plan your meals ahead of time and shop accordingly, filling your kitchen with keto-friendly foods.

Healthy snacks

To make it easier to stick to the keto diet, it's important to have healthy snacks. If you're on the keto diet with your partner, have keto-approved snacks on hand that you both enjoy. Approved snacks include:

- Hard-boiled eggs, cheese, and olives
- A handful of nuts and seeds
- Celery and red pepper sticks with guacamole and salsa
- No-sugar plain yogurt mixed with berries

Intermittent Fasting and the Keto Diet

Intermittent fasting is all about restricting the number of calories you consume within a period so that you put your body into a "fasted" state. When this happens, the body's insulin levels will start to lower, which increases the fat burning process.

The Benefits of Intermittent Fasting Include:

- Weight loss
- Improved mental clarity
- Management and reducing the risk of type 2 diabetes
- Lower risk of cardiovascular disease
- Lower risk of some cancers

The most common fasting method is to fast each day for 14 to 16 hours, restricting the time you eat to a "window" of 8 to 10 hours. During the eating window, you should be eating at least 2 to 3 healthy keto meals. An excellent way to approach intermittent fasting is eating your last meal by 8 pm on any day and not eating your first meal until midnight the next day.

Another intermittent fasting method includes the 5:2 rule, where you only eat 500 to 600 calories per day on two days of the week, eating a healthy keto diet for the other five days. Another fasting method is the eat-stop-eat plan, where you fast for 24 hours twice a week.

Both intermittent fasting and the keto diet put the body into a ketosis state to use up stored fat for energy. When you combine intermittent fasting with the keto diet, you may be able to put your body into ketosis faster than dieting alone. This can lead to faster and more efficient weight loss.

What to Expect On the Keto Diet & Keto "Flu"

During the first few days of starting the Keto, you may experience an increase in hunger, lack of energy, and problems sleeping. Some people may also experience nausea and digestive issues. These flu-like symptoms are known as the "keto flu." To alleviate these symptoms, consider doing a low-carb diet for a week slowly transitioning into the full keto diet. During the first month, always eat until you feel full without focusing on restricting calories. Ease into the food plan, so you're less likely to stop eating a ketogenic diet.

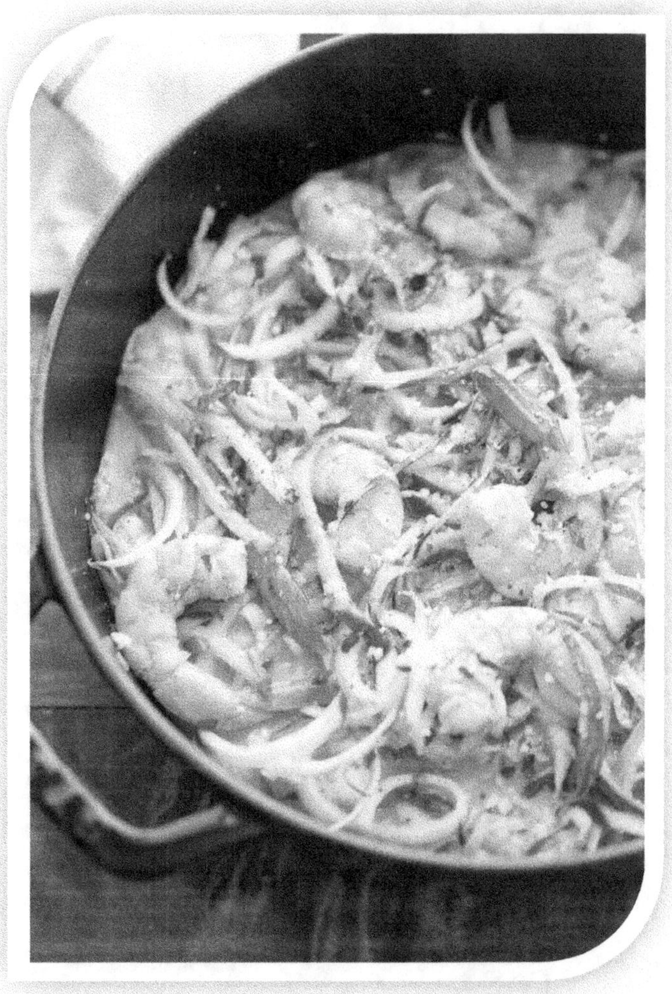

The keto diet changes the mineral and water balance of your body. Make sure that you're drinking more water each day. As well, taking a mineral supplement and adding a bit of extra salt to your diet can keep help maintain a healthy balance of minerals and water, helping to relieve any of the flu-like symptoms. For a mineral supplement, take 300 mg of magnesium and 1,000 mg of potassium.

DIET – THE NEW LIFESTYLE

The Benefits of Keto Diet

Even though it is still considered 'controversial,' the keto diet is the best dietary choice one can make. From weight loss to longevity, here are the benefits that following a ketogenic diet can bring to your life:

Loss of Appetite

You can't tame your cravings? Don't worry. While on ketosis, you won't feel exhausted or with a rumbling gut. The keto diet will help you say no to that second piece of cake. Once you train your body to run on fat and not on carbs, you will experience a drop in appetite that will work magic for your figure.

Weight Loss

Since the body is forced to produce only a small amount of glucose, it will lower insulin production. When that happens, your kidneys will start getting rid of the extra sodium, which will lead to weight loss.

HDL Cholesterol Increase and Drop in Blood Pressure

While consuming a diet high in fat and staying clear of harmful glucose, your body will experience a rise in good HDL cholesterol levels, which will, in turn, reduce the risk for many cardiovascular problems. Cutting back on carbs will also drop your blood pressure. The drop in blood pressure can prevent many health problems such as strokes or heart diseases.

Lower Risk of Diabetes

Although this probably goes without saying, it is essential to mention this one. When you ditch the carbs, your body is forced to lower the glucose productivity significantly, which leads to a lower risk of diabetes, including a reverse in the condition if you already have it.

Improved Brain Function

Many studies have shown that replacing carbohydrates with fat as an energy source leads to mental clarity and improved brain function. This is yet another reason why you should go Keto.

Should You Try the Keto Diet?

The keto diet can help you lose weight and keep it off. When you're eating nutritiously, exercising, and following a ketogenic food plan, you'll be joining the many other people around the world who have successfully lost weight.

Whether you're starting the keto diet on your own or as a couple, begin with the keto food plan basics to become familiar with the foods you can and can't eat. As you start to lose weight and learn how to customize your meals, the keto diet plan will become a natural part of your lifestyle, allowing you to maintain your health and weight loss.

BASIC & SIMPLE RECIPES

1.HOMEMADE GUACAMOLE

Ingredients

- For 4 servings
- 2 avocados, peeled, pitted
- ½ yellow onion, minced
- ½ lime, juiced
- 1 tomato, peeled, chopped
- 2 tbsp fresh cilantro, chopped
- Salt and chili powder to taste

Directions

1. Total Time: approx. 10 minutes
2. Mash the avocado with a fork in a bowl.
3. Mix in the onion, lime juice, tomato, chili powder, and salt.
4. Sprinkle with cilantro and serve immediately.

Per serving:

- Cal 173
- Net Carbs 1.4g
- Fat 15.8g
- Protein 2g

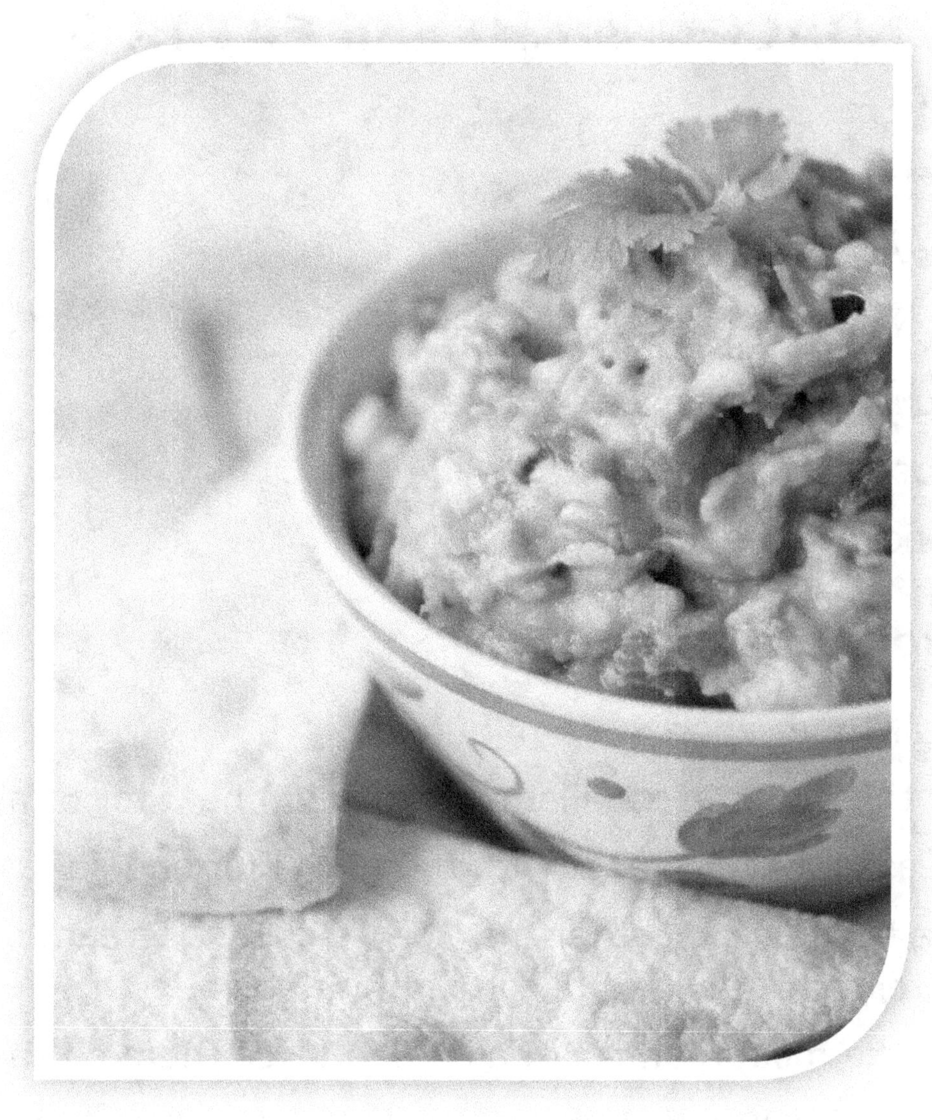

2.BACON & CHEESE FAT BOMB

Ingredients

For 3 servings (6 fat bombs)

- ¼ cup Chèvre cheese, grated
- ¼ cup cream cheese, softened
- 2 tbsp butter, softened
- 4 bacon slices, chopped

Directions

1. Total Time: approx. 45 minutes
2. Fry the bacon in a skillet over medium heat for 5 minutes.
3. Grease a baking sheet with the bacon fat and set aside.
4. In a bowl, stir together the Chèvre cheese, cream cheese, butter, and stir-fried bacon until well blended.
5. Roll the mixture into 8 "balls" and place them on the sheet.
6. Freeze for 30 minutes.

Per serving:

- Cal 282
- Net Carbs 0.1g
- Fat 26g
- Protein 11 g

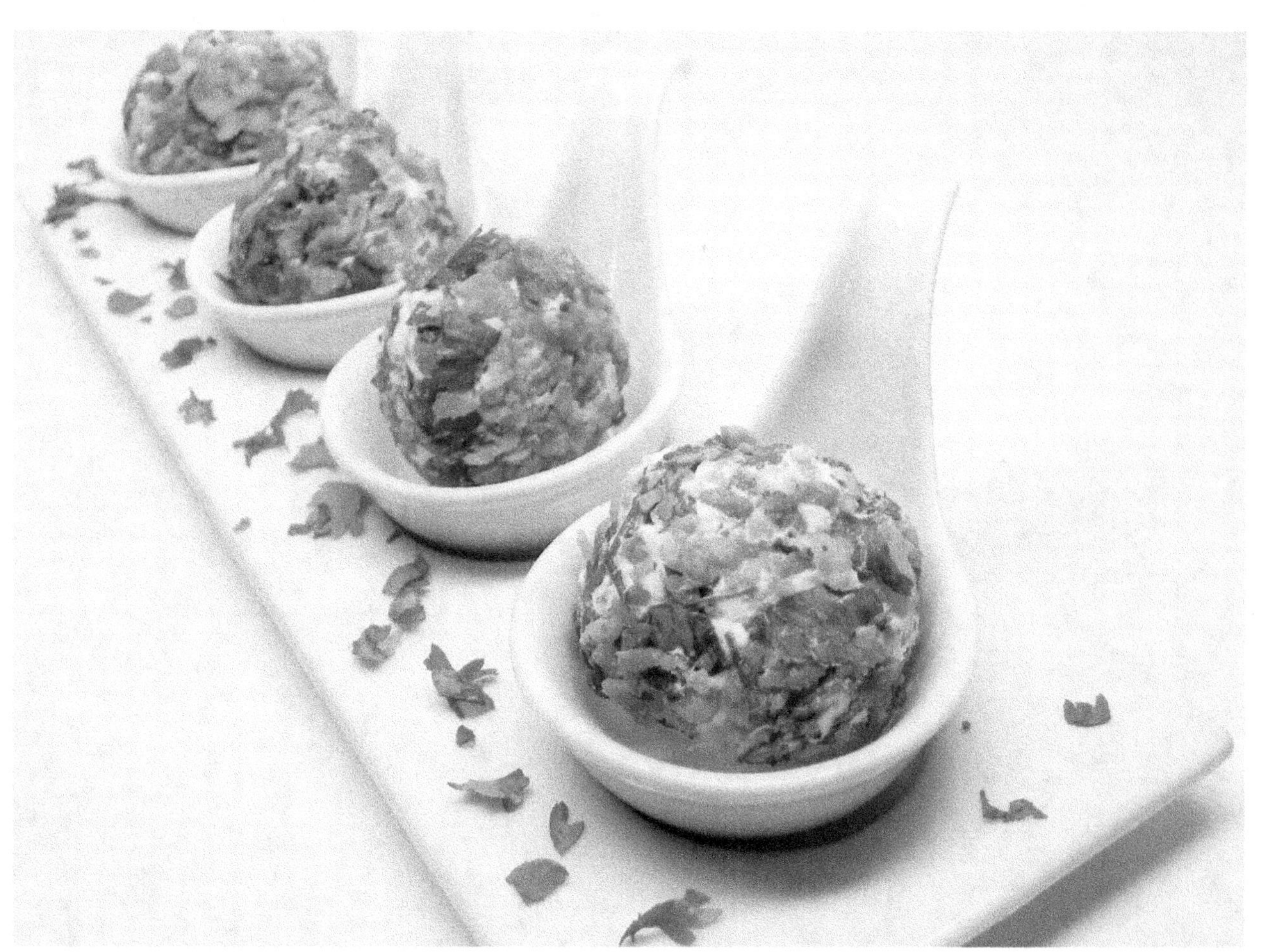

BREAKFAST & EGGS

3. CRESPELLE AL MASCARPONE

Ingredients

For 2 servings

- ½ cup almond flour
- 2 tsp liquid stevia
- 1 tsp baking powder
- ½ cup almond milk
- 1 tsp vanilla extract
- 1 large egg
- ¼ cup olive oil
- Whole raspberries to garnish
- 1 cup mascarpone cheese
- 1 tsp mint, chopped

Directions

Total Time: approx. 35 minutes

1. Beat the egg in a bowl.
2. Add in the almond milk, vanilla extract, and half of the stevia and stir to combine.
3. In another bowl, whisk the almond flour and baking powder together.
4. Then, pour the egg mixture into the almond flour mixture and continue whisking until smooth.
5. Heat olive oil in a pan over medium heat and pour in 1 soup spoon of batter.

6. Cook on one side for 2 minutes, flip the pancake, and cook the other side for 2 minutes.

7. Transfer the pancake to a plate and repeat the cooking process until the batter is exhausted.

8. Mix the mascarpone with the remaining stevia and mint in a small bowl.

9. Spread each mini pancake with mascarpone and scatter raspberry over to serve.

Per serving:

- Cal 687
- Fat 61g
- Net Carbs 5.2g
- Protein 23g

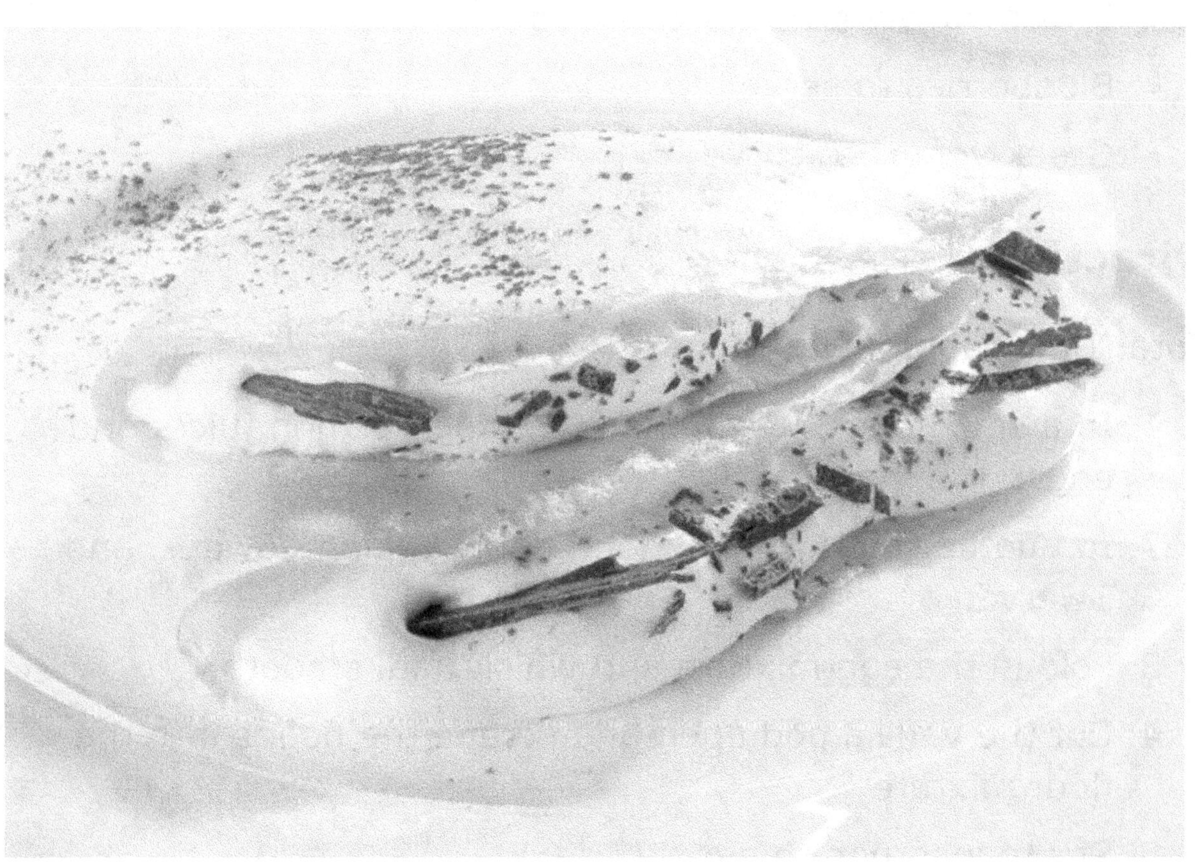

4. PERFECT BUTTERMILK PANCAKES

Ingredients

For 4 servings

- 3 eggs
- ½ cup buttermilk
- ½ cup almond flour
- ½ tsp baking powder
- 1 tbsp Swerve
- 1 lemon, juiced
- 1 vanilla pod
- 2 tbsp unsalted butter
- 2 tbsp olive oil
- 3 tbsp sugar- free maple syrup
- Blueberries to serve
- Greek yogurt to serve

Directions

Total Time: approx. 25 minutes

1. In a small bowl, whisk the buttermilk, lemon juice, and eggs.
2. In another bowl, mix almond flour, baking powder, and Swerve.
3. Fold in the egg mixture and whisk until smooth.
4. Cut the vanilla pod open and scrape the beans into the flour mixture.
5. Stir to incorporate evenly.

6. In a skillet, melt a quarter of the butter and olive oil and spoon in 2 tablespoons of the pancake mixture into the pan.

7. Cook for 4 minutes or until small bubbles appear.

8. Flip and cook for 2 minutes or until set and golden.

9. Repeat the cooking until the batter finishes using the remaining butter and olive oil in the same proportions.

10. Plate the pancakes, drizzle with maple syrup, top with a generous dollop of yogurt, and scatter some blueberries on top.

Per serving:

- Cal 172
- Net Carbs 1.6g
- Fat 12g
- Protein 7g

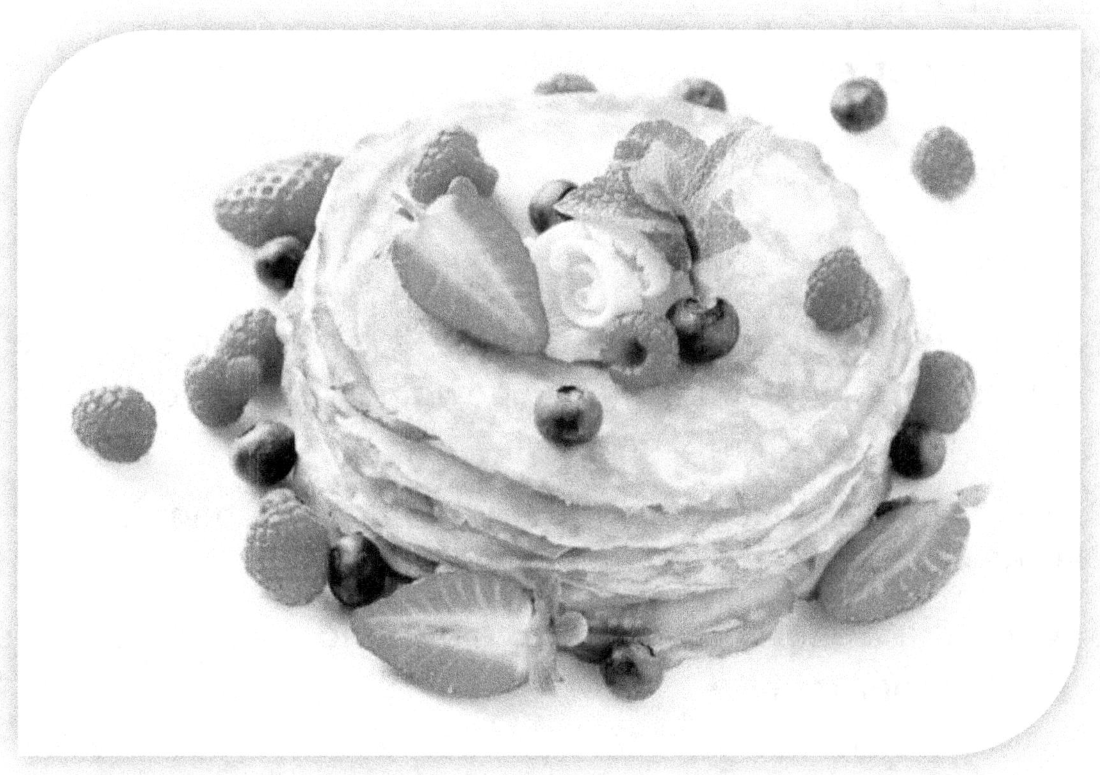

5. GINGER PANCAKES

Ingredients

For 2 servings

- 1 cup almond flour
- 1 tsp cinnamon powder
- 2 tbsp Swerve
- ¼ tsp baking soda
- 1 tsp ginger powder
- 1 egg
- 1 cup almond milk
- 2 tbsp olive oil **Lime sauce**
- ¼ cup liquid stevia
- ½ tsp arrowroot starch
- ½ lime, juiced and zested
- 2 tbsp butter

Directions

Total Time: approx. 20 minutes

1. Combine together the almond flour, cinnamon powder, Swerve, baking soda, ginger powder, egg, almond milk, and olive oil in a mixing bowl.

2. Heat oil in a skillet over medium heat and spoon 2-3 tablespoons of the mixture into the skillet.

3. Cook the batter for 1 minute, flip it and cook the other side for another minute.

4. Remove the pancake onto a plate and repeat the cooking process until the batter is exhausted.

5. Mix the stevia and arrowroot starch in a saucepan.

6. Set the pan over medium heat and gradually stir 1 cup water until it thickens, about 1 minute.

7. Turn the heat off and add the butter, lime juice, and lime zest.

8. Stir the mixture until the butter melts.

9. Drizzle the sauce over the pancakes and serve warm.

Per serving:

- Cal 343
- Fat 25g
- Net Carbs 6.1g
- Protein 8g

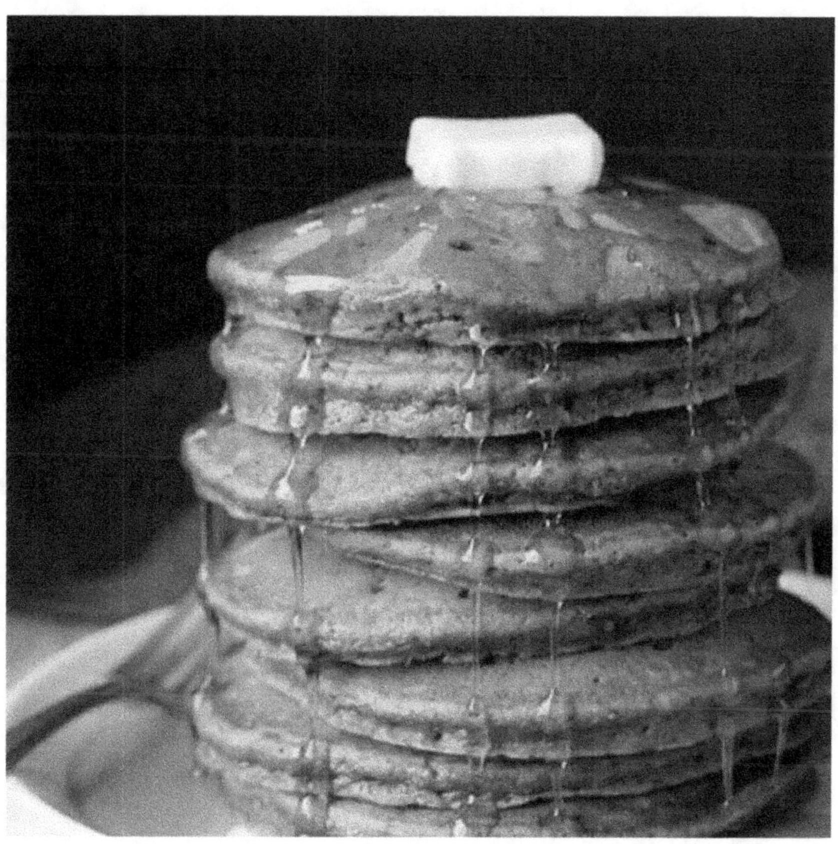

SALADS & SOUPS

6. SAUSAGE & PESTO SALAD WITH CHEESE

Ingredients

For 2 servings

- ½ cup mixed cherry tomatoes, cut in half
- ½ lb pork sausage links, sliced
- 1 cups mixed lettuce greens
- ¼ cup radicchio, sliced
- 1 tbsp olive oil
- ¼ lb feta cheese, cubed
- ½ tbsp lemon juice
- ¼ cup basil pesto
- 6 black olives, pitted, halved
- Salt and black pepper, to taste
- 1 tbsp Parmesan shavings

Directions

Total Time: approx. 10 minutes

1. Cook the sausages in warm olive oil over medium heat for 5-6 minutes, stirring often.
2. In a salad bowl, combine the mixed lettuce greens, radicchio, feta cheese, pesto, cherry tomatoes, black olives, and lemon juice and toss well to coat.
3. Season with salt and black pepper and add the sausages.
4. Sprinkle with Parmesan shavings and serve.

Per serving:

- Cal 611
- Fat 48g
- Net Carbs 7.5g
- Protein 31g

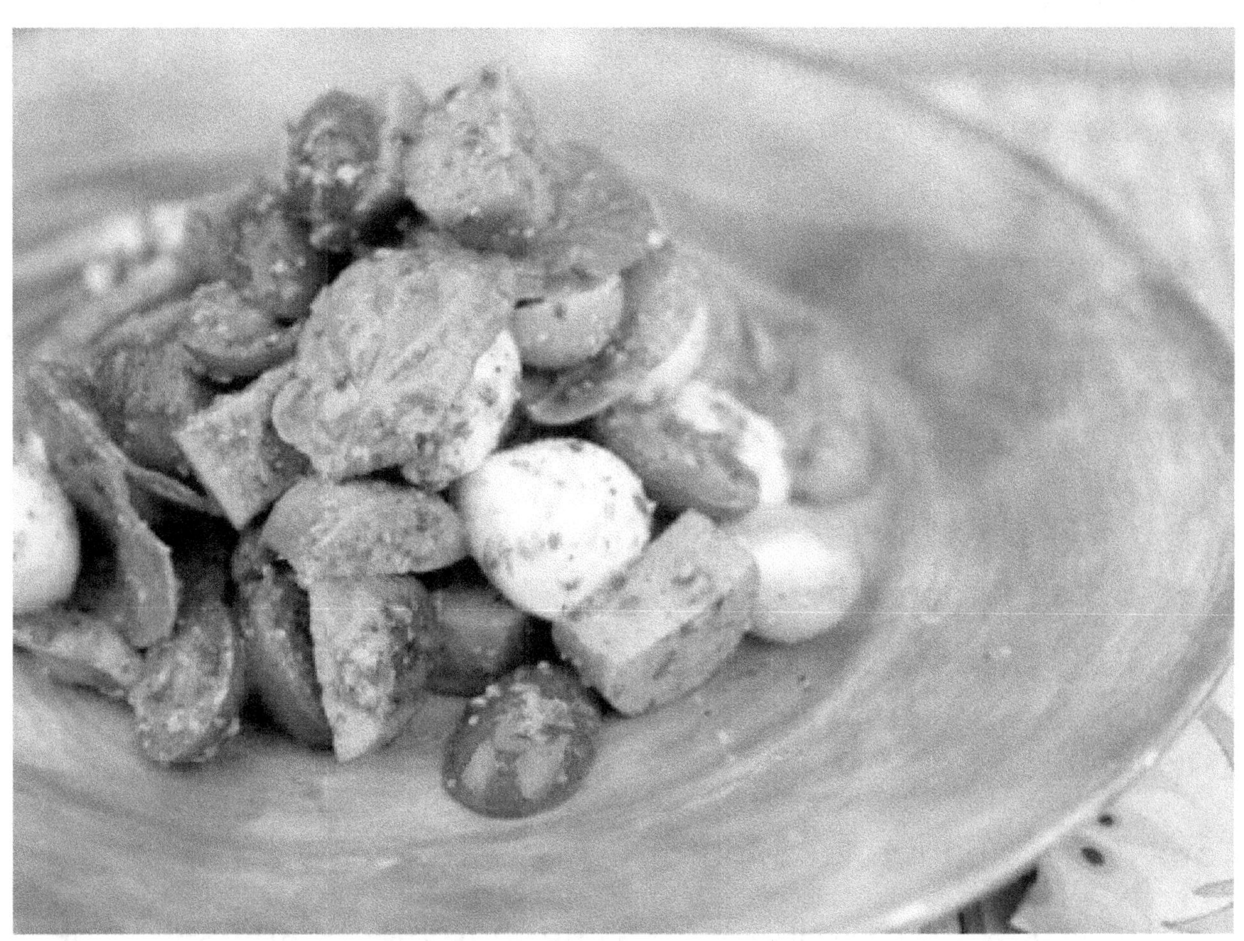

7. SMOKED SALMON, BACON & EGG SALAD

Ingredients

For 4 servings

- 1 eggs
- 1 head romaine lettuce, torn
- 4 oz smoked salmon, chopped
- 3 slices bacon
- 4 cherry tomatoes, halved Salt and black pepper to taste

Dressing:

- ½ cup mayonnaise
- ½ tsp garlic puree
- 1 tbsp lemon juice
- 1 tsp tabasco sauce

Directions

Total Time: approx. 20 minutes

1. In a bowl, mix well the dressing ingredients and set aside.
2. Bring a pot of salted water to a boil.
3. Crack each egg into a small bowl and gently slide into the water.
4. Poach for 2-3 minutes.
5. Remove with a perforated spoon, transfer to a paper towel to dry, and plate.

6. Put the bacon in a skillet over medium heat and fry until browned and crispy, about 6 minutes, turning once.

7. Remove, allow cooling, and chop into small pieces.

8. Toss the lettuce, smoked salmon, bacon, and dressing in a salad bowl.

9. Divide the salad between plates, top with the eggs each, and serve immediately or chilled.

Per serving:

- Cal 291
- Fat 19g
- Net Carbs 6.4g
- Protein 15g

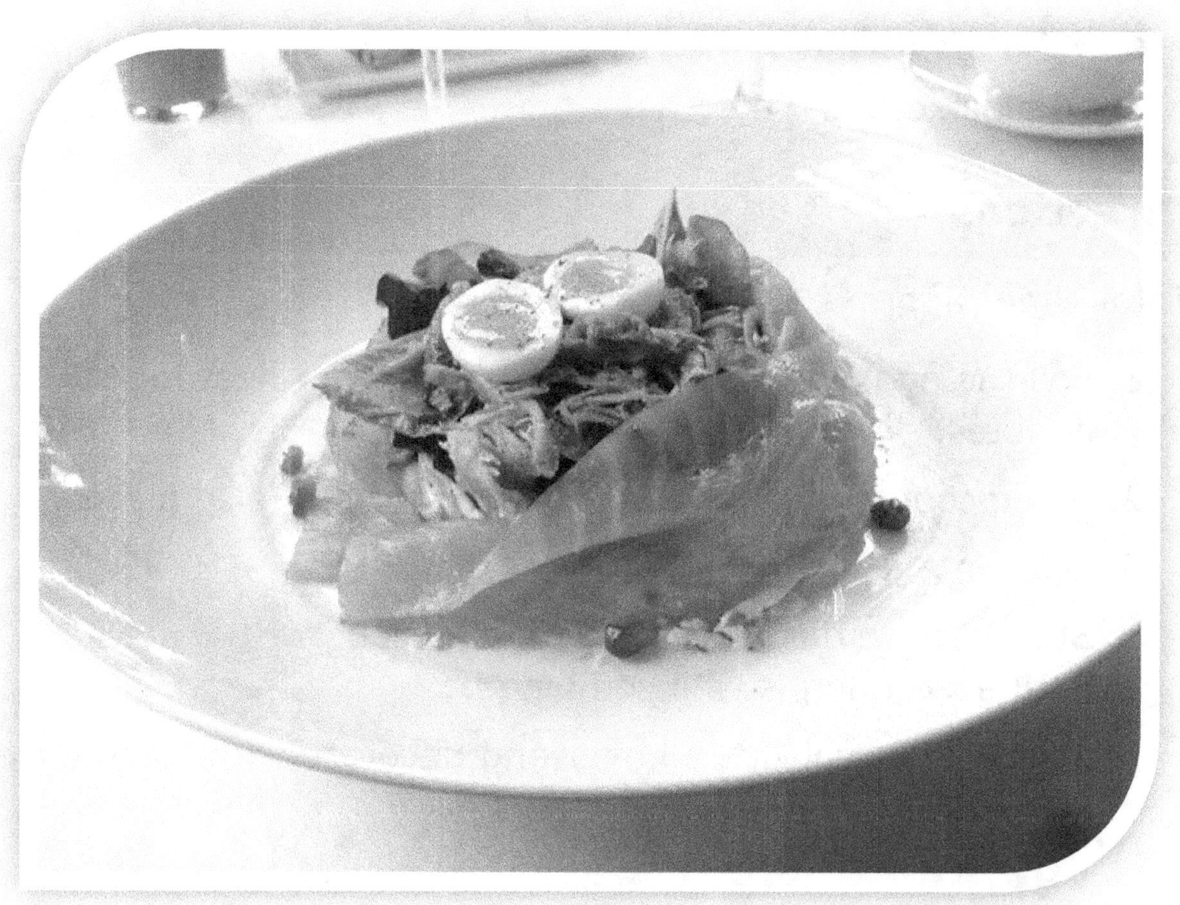

8. CLASSIC EGG SALAD WITH OLIVES

Ingredients

For 2 servings

- 4 eggs
- ¼ cup mayonnaise
- ½ tsp sriracha sauce
- ½ tbsp mustard
- ¼ cup scallions
- ¼ stalk celery, minced
- Salt and black pepper, to taste
- 1 head romaine lettuce, torn
- ¼ tsp fresh lime juice
- 10 black olives

Directions

Total Time: approx. 15 minutes

1. Boil the eggs in salted water over medium heat for 10 minutes.
2. When cooled, peel and chop them into bite-size pieces.
3. Place in a salad bowl.
4. Stir in the remaining ingredients, except for the scallions, until everything is well combined.
5. Scatter the scallions all over and decorate with black olives to serve.

Per serving:

- Cal 312
- Fat 22g
- Net Carbs 6.3g
- Protein 17g

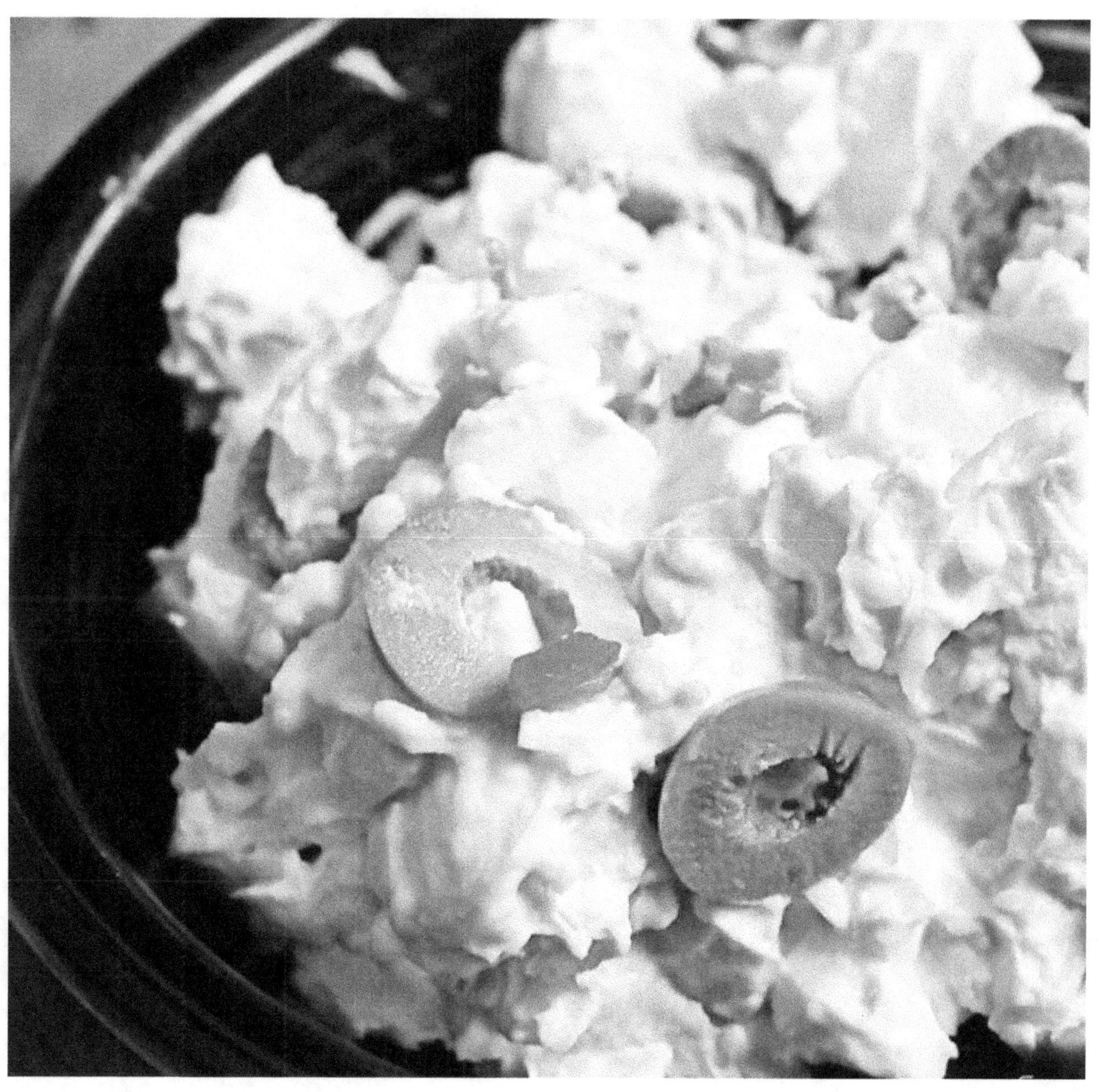

POULTRY

9. BAKED CHICKEN NUGGETS

Ingredients

For 2 servings

- 2 tbsp ranch dressing
- ½ cup almond flour
- 1 egg
- 2 tbsp garlic powder
- 2 chicken breasts, cubed
- Salt and black pepper, to taste
- 1 tbsp butter, melted

Directions

Total Time: approx. 30 minutes

1. Preheat oven to 400 F.
2. Grease a baking dish with butter.
3. In a bowl, combine salt, garlic powder, almond flour, and black pepper and stir.
4. In a separate bowl, beat the egg.
5. Dredge the chicken cubes to the egg, then in the flour mixture.
6. Cook in the oven for 18-20 minutes, turning halfway through, until golden and crispy.
7. Remove to paper towels, drain the excess grease and serve with ranch dressing, if desired.

Per serving:

- Cal 473
- Fat 31g
- Net Carbs 7.6g
- Protein 43g

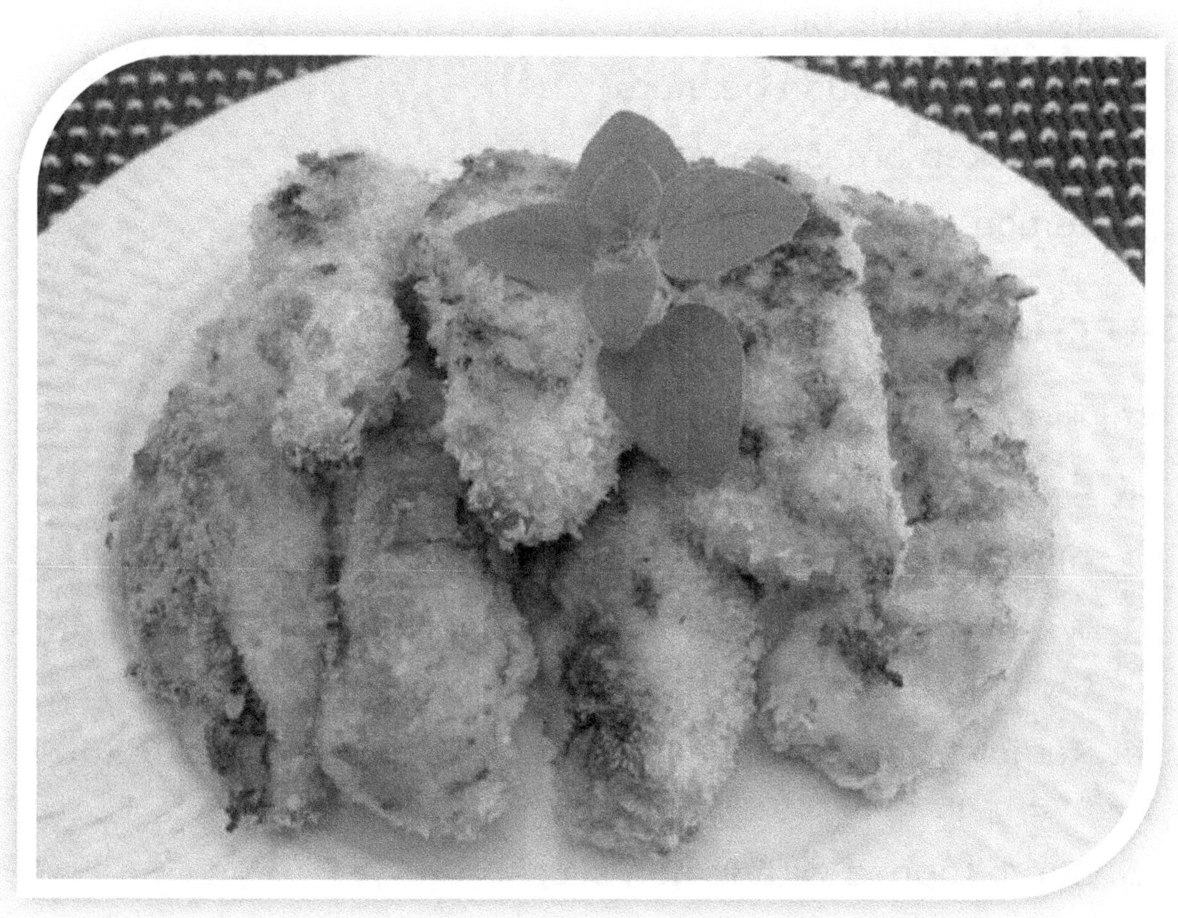

10. PEANUT-CRUSTED CHICKEN

Ingredients

For 2 servings

- 1 egg, beaten
- Salt and black pepper to taste
- 3 tbsp canola oil
- 1 ½ cups ground peanuts
- 2 chicken breast halves
- Lemon slices for garnish

Directions

Total Time: approx. 25 minutes

1. Season the chicken with salt and pepper.
2. Dip in the egg and then in ground peanuts.
3. Warm the canola oil in a pan over medium heat and brown the chicken for 2 minutes per side.
4. Remove to a baking sheet, set in the preheated to 360 F oven, and bake for 10 minutes.
5. Serve topped with lemon slices.

Per serving:

- Cal 634
- Fat 51g
- Net Carbs 4.7g
- Protein 46g

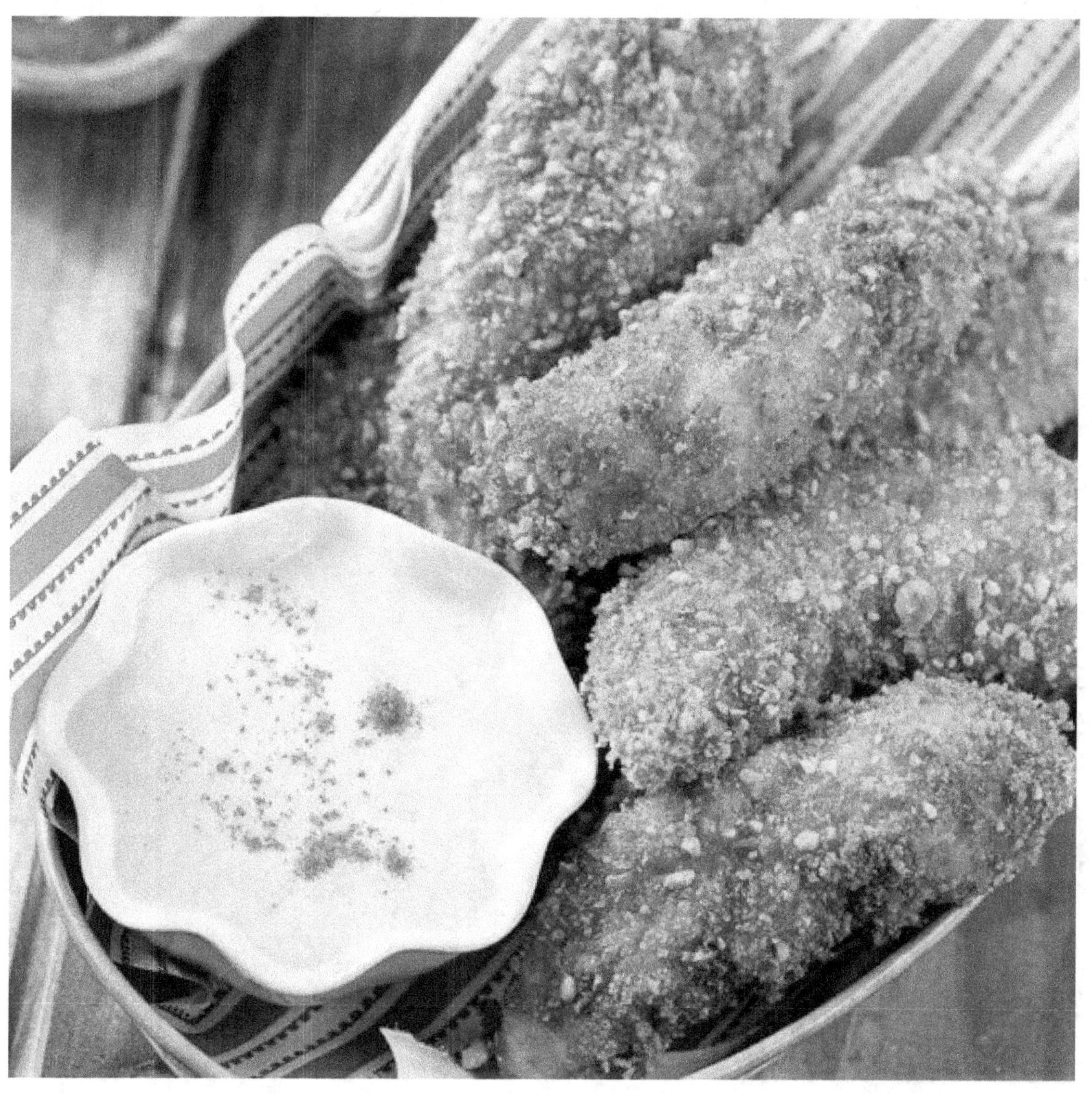

11.CHICKEN DIPPERS WITH HOMEMADE KETCHUP

Ingredients

For 4 servings

- 1 lb chicken breasts, cut into strips
- 14 oz canned tomatoes, diced
- 1 tbsp tomato paste
- ½ tbsp xylitol
- 1 tbsp balsamic vinegar
- 1 cup tomato sauce
- 1 tbsp basil, chopped
- ½ cup almond flour
- ¼ cup Parmesan, grated
- ½ tsp garlic powder
- 1 tsp dried parsley
- ½ tsp dried thyme
- Salt and black pepper to taste
- 1 egg, beaten in a bowl
- 2 tbsp olive oil

Directions

Total Time: approx. 35 minutes

1. Place a saucepan over medium heat. Add the tomatoes, tomato paste, xylitol, tomato sauce, salt, pepper, and balsamic vinegar and bring to a boil. Cook for 10-15

minutes, stirring frequently until thickened. Adjust the seasoning. Top the ketchup with basil and set aside.

2. In a bowl, combine the almond flour, parsley, Parmesan, pepper, garlic powder, thyme, and salt. Dip the chicken strips in the egg and then in the almond flour mixture.

3. Heat a pan over medium heat and warm the olive oil. Fry the chicken until golden, about 4-6 minutes. Remove to paper towels to soak the excess oil. Serve with ketchup.

Per serving:

- Cal 336
- Fat 21g
- Net Carbs 7.7g
- Protein 25g

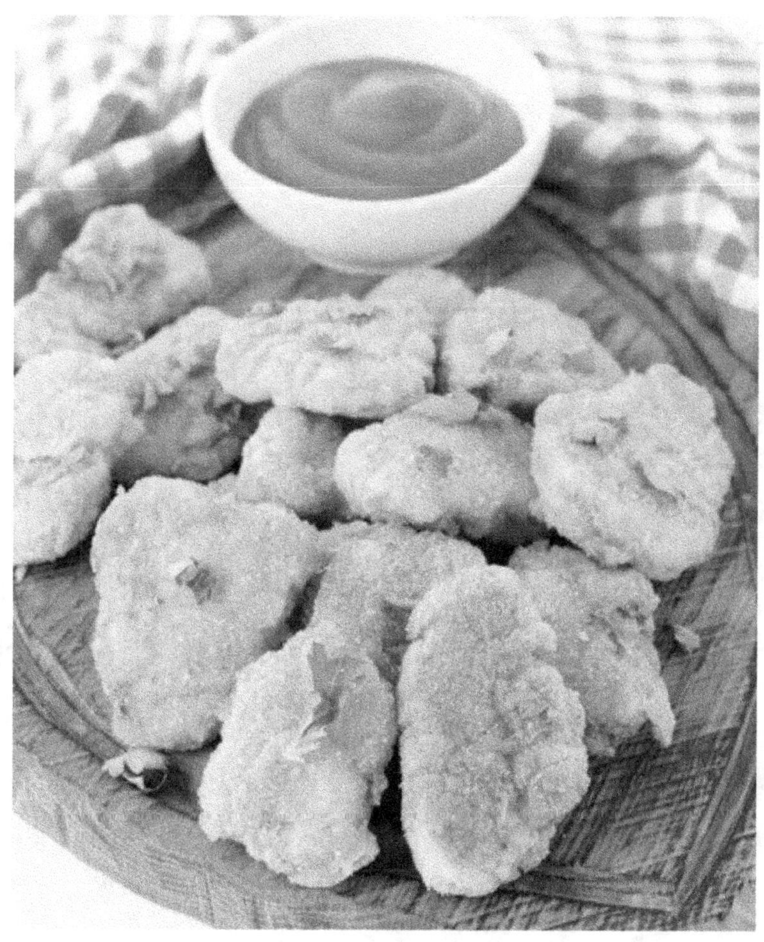

12. WINTER CHICKEN WITH VEGETABLES

Ingredients

For 2 servings

- 2 tbsp olive oil
- 2 cups whipping cream
- 1 lb chicken breasts, chopped
- 1 onion, chopped
- 1 carrot, chopped
- 2 cups chicken stock
- Salt and black pepper, to taste
- 1 bay leaf
- 1 turnip, chopped
- 1 parsnip, chopped
- 1 cup green beans, chopped
- 2 tsp fresh thyme, chopped

Directions

Total Time: approx. 40 minutes

1. Heat a pan over medium heat and warm the olive oil.
2. Sauté the onion for 3 minutes, pour in the stock, carrot, turnip, parsnip, chicken, and bay leaf.
3. Bring to a boil and simmer for 20 minutes.
4. Add in the green beans and cook for 7 minutes.

5. Discard the bay leaf, stir in the whipping cream, adjust the taste and scatter with thyme to serve.

Per serving:

- Cal 483
- Fat 32g
- Net Carbs 6.9g
- Protein 33g

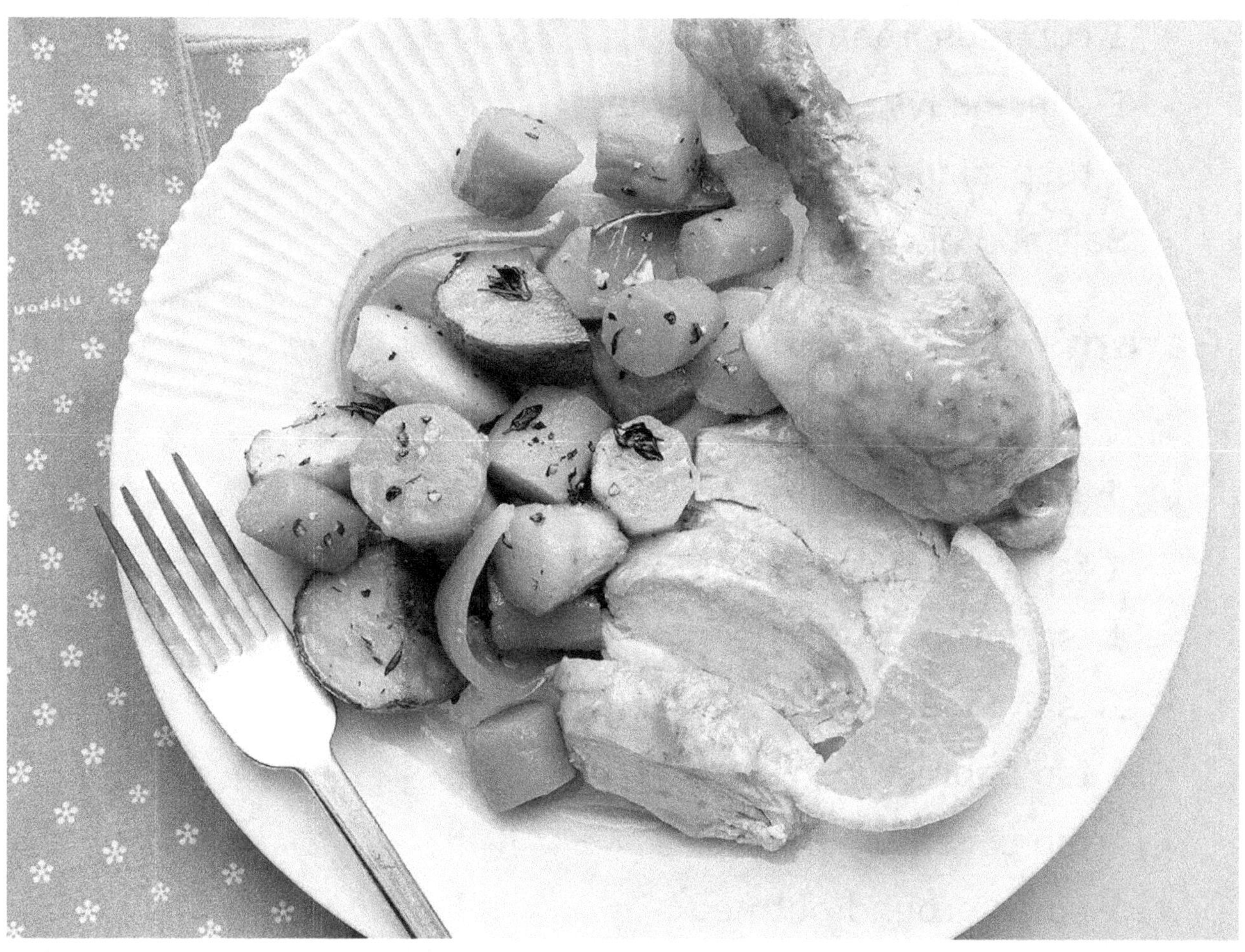

13. INDIAN CHICKEN WITH MUSHROOMS

Ingredients

For 4 servings

- 1 lb chicken breasts, sliced lengthwise
- 2 tbsp butter
- 1 tbsp olive oil
- 1 cup mushrooms
- 2 cups heavy whipping cream
- 1 tbsp cilantro, chopped
- Salt and black pepper to taste

Garam masala

- 1 tsp ground cumin
- 2 tsp ground coriander
- 1 tsp ground cardamom
- 1 tsp turmeric
- 1 tsp ginger
- 1 tsp paprika
- 1 tsp cayenne, ground
- 1 pinch ground nutmeg

Directions

Total Time: approx. 35 minutes

1 Preheat oven to 370 F.

2 In a bowl, mix all the garam masala spices.

3 Coat the chicken with the mixture.

4 Heat the olive oil and butter in a frying pan over medium heat, and brown the chicken for 3-5 minutes per side.

5 Transfer to a baking dish.

6 In a bowl, mix the heavy cream and mushrooms.

7 Season with salt and pepper and pour over the chicken.

8 Bake for 20 minutes until the mixture starts to bubble.

9 Garnish with chopped cilantro to serve.

Per serving:

- Cal 553
- Fat 49g
- Net Carbs 4.5g
- Protein 32g

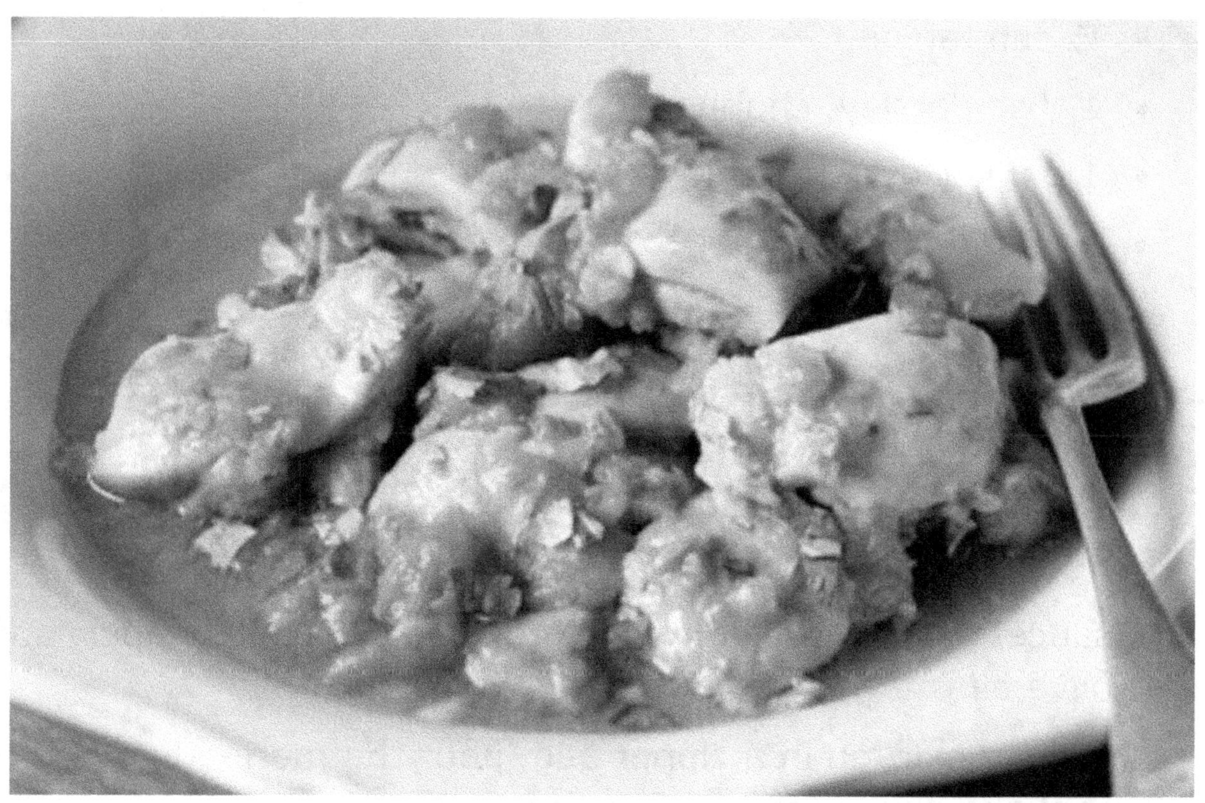

14. CHILI CHICKEN KEBAB WITH GARLIC DRESSING

Ingredients

For 4 servings

Skewers

- 2 tbsp olive oil
- 3 tbsp soy sauce, sugar- free
- 1 tbsp ginger paste
- 2 tbsp Swerve brown sugar
- 2 Chili pepper to taste
- 2 chicken breasts, cubed

Dressing

- ½ cup tahini
- 1 tbsp parsley, chopped
- 1 garlic clove, minced
- Salt and black pepper to taste
- ¼ cup warm water

Directions

Total Time: approx. 25 min + cooling time

1. To make the marinade, in a small bowl, whisk the soy sauce, ginger paste, Swerve brown sugar, chili pepper, and olive oil.

2. Put the chicken in a zipper bag, pour the marinade over, seal and shake for an even coat.

3 Marinate in the fridge for 2 hours.

4 Preheat a grill to high heat.

5 Thread the chicken on skewers and cook for 10 minutes in total with three to four turnings to be golden brown.

6 Transfer to a plate.

7 Mix the dressing ingredients in a bowl.

8 Serve the chicken skewers topped with the tahini dressing.

Per serving:

- Cal 410

- Fat 32g

- Net Carbs 4.8g

- Protein 23g

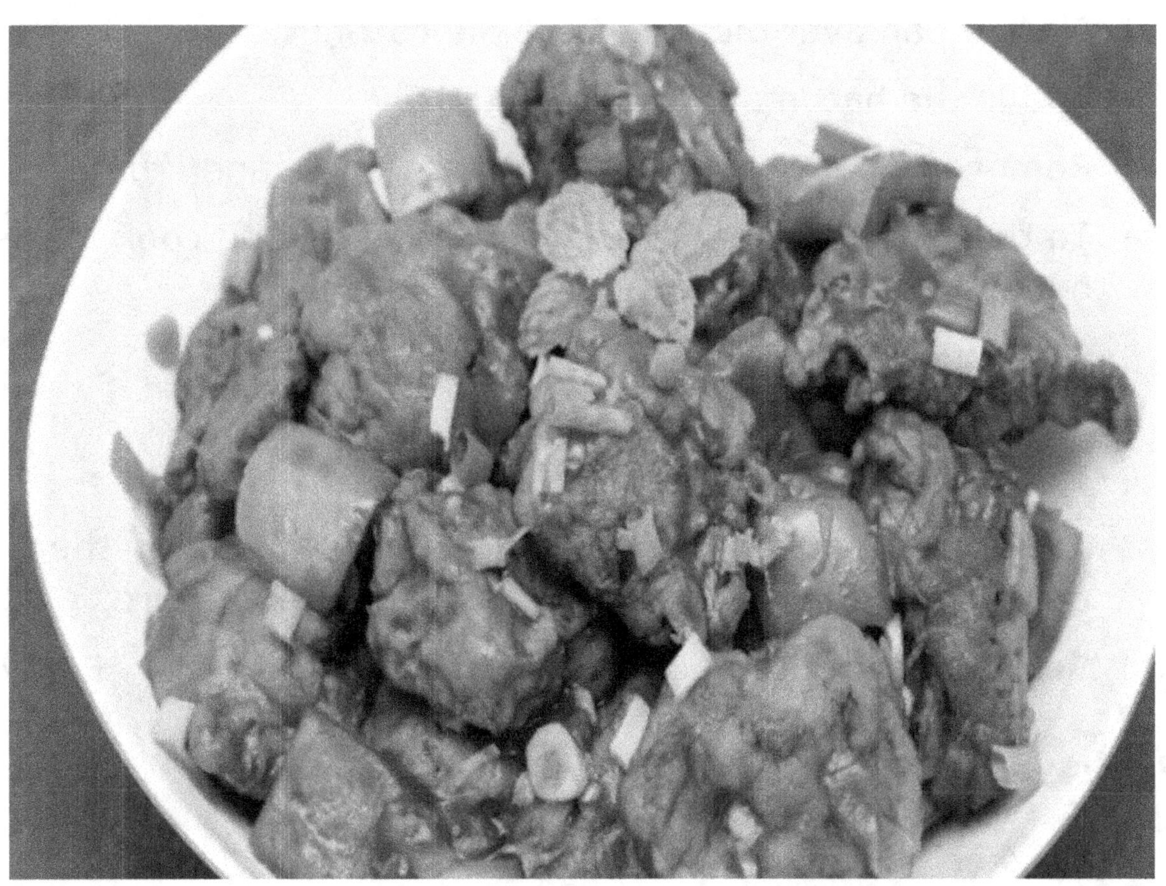

15. FETA & BACON CHICKEN

Ingredients

For 4 servings

- 4 oz bacon, chopped
- 1 lb chicken breasts
- 3 green onions, chopped
- 2 tbsp coconut oil
- 4 oz feta cheese, crumbled
- 1 tbsp parsley

Directions

Total Time: approx. 25 minutes

1. Place a pan over medium heat the coconut oil.
2. Add in the bacon and cook until crispy.
3. Remove to paper towels, drain the grease, and crumble.
4. To the same pan, add the chicken breasts and cook for 4-5 minutes.
5. Flip to the other side and cook for an additional 4-5 minutes.
6. Transfer to a baking dish.
7. Top with the green onions, set in the oven, turn on the broiler, and cook for 5 minutes at high temperature.
8. Serve topped with bacon, feta cheese, and parsley. Enjoy!

Per serving:

- Cal 459

- Fat 35g
- Net Carbs 3.1g
- Protein 32g

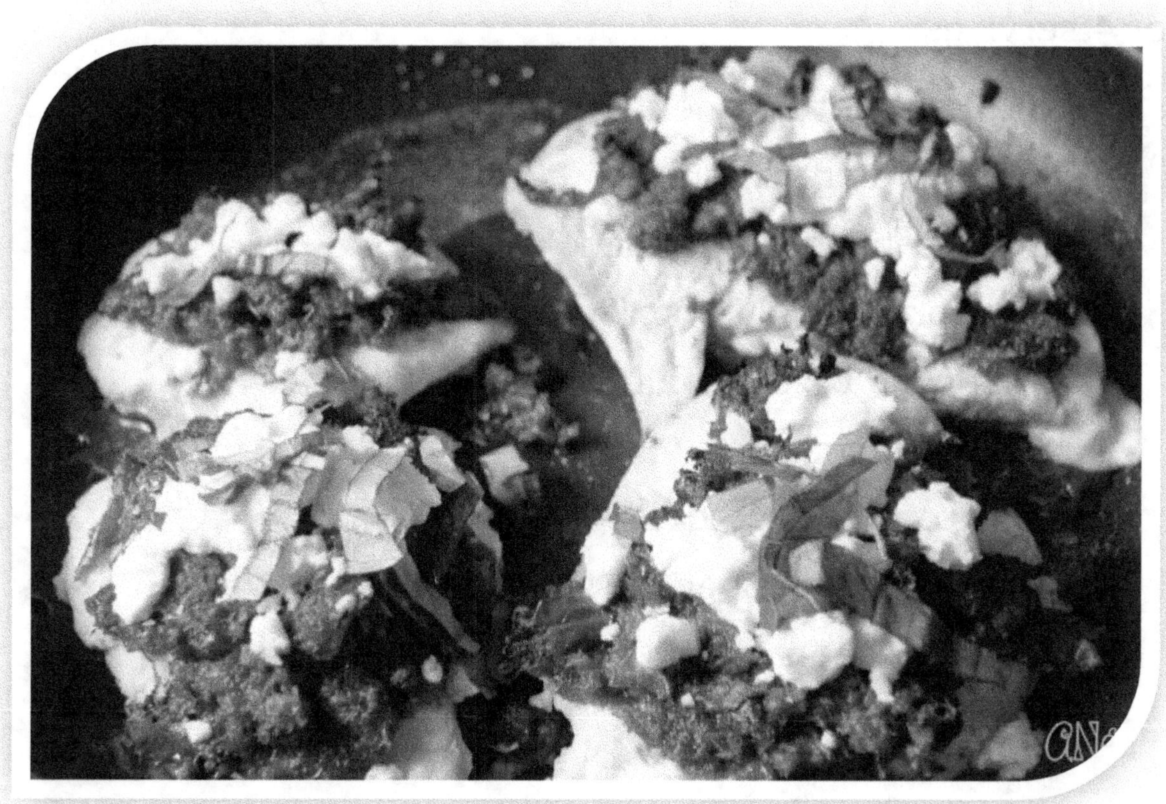

16. CABBAGE & BROCCOLI CHICKEN CASSEROLE

Ingredients

For 4 servings

- 1 tbsp coconut oil, melted
- 2 cups mozzarella, grated
- ½ head cabbage, shredded
- 1 head broccoli, cut into florets
- 1 lb chicken breasts, cubed
- 1 cup mayonnaise
- 1 /3 cup chicken stock
- Salt and black pepper, to taste
- Juice of 1 lemon
- 1 tbsp cilantro, chopped

Directions

Total Time: approx. 60 minutes

1　Coat a baking dish with coconut oil and set chicken pieces to the bottom.
2　Top with the green cabbage and broccoli and sprinkle with half of mozzarella cheese.
3　In a bowl, combine the mayonnaise with black pepper, stock, lemon juice, and salt.
4　Spread the mixture over the chicken, top with the rest of the mozzarella cheese, and cover with aluminum foil.
5　Bake for 30 minutes in the oven at 350 F.

6 Open aluminum foil and cook for 20 more minutes.

7 Sprinkle with cilantro and serve.

Per serving:

- Cal 623
- Fat 42g
- Net Carbs 7.4g
- Protein 52g

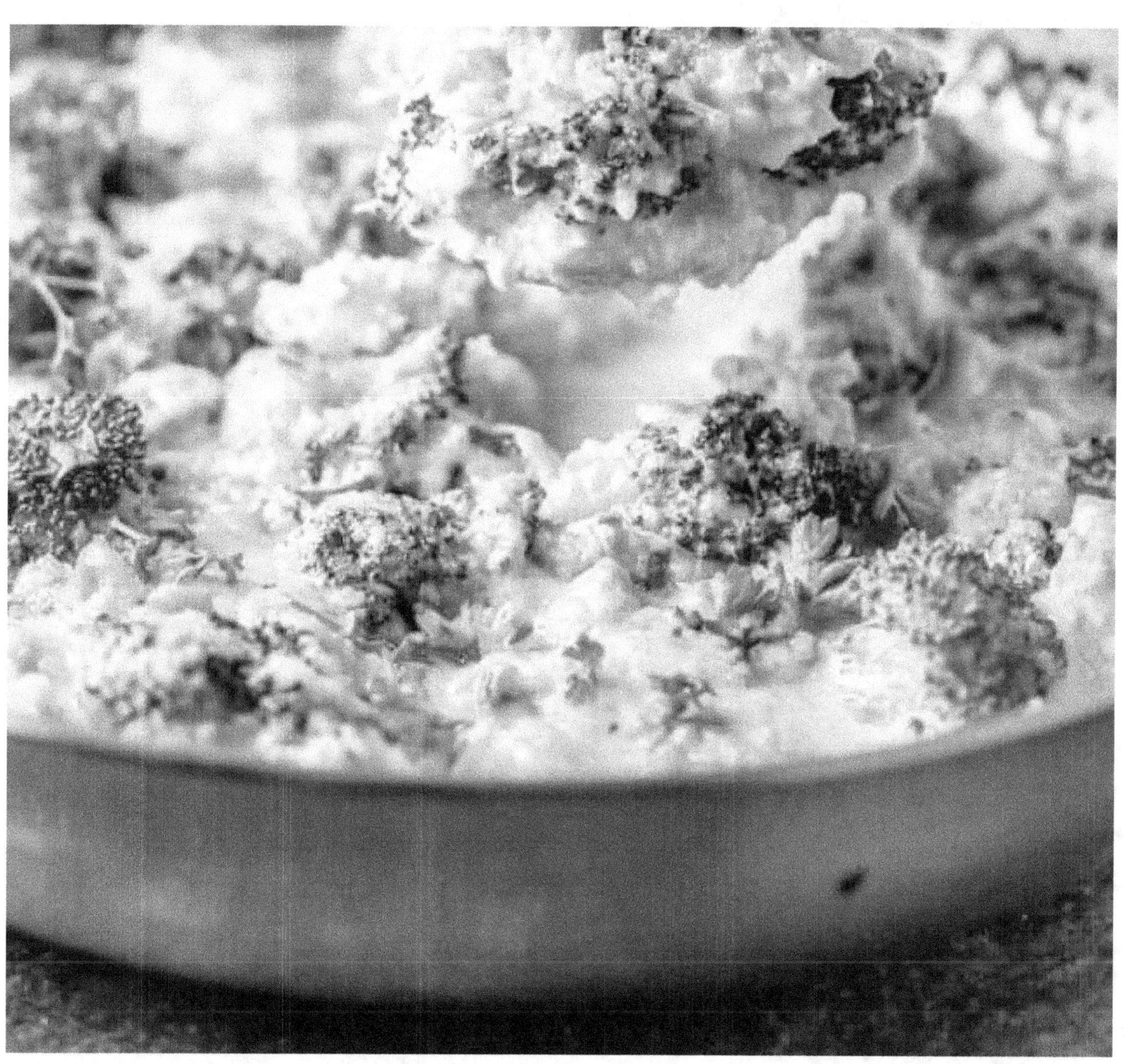

17. FENNEL & CHICKEN WRAPPED IN BACON

Ingredients

For 4 servings

- 2 tbsp olive oil
- 2 chicken breasts
- Salt and black pepper to taste
- 4 bacon slices
- ½ lb fennel bulb, sliced
- 2 tbsp lemon juice
- 2 tbsp cheddar cheese, grated
- 1 tbsp rosemary, chopped

Directions

Total Time: approx. 50 minutes

1. Preheat your grill to high heat.
2. Brush the fennel slices with olive oil and season with salt and black pepper.
3. Grill for 4-6 minutes, frequently turning until slightly golden.
4. Remove to a plate and drizzle with lemon juice.
5. Pour over cheddar cheese so that it melts a little on contact with the hot fennel and forms a cheesy dressing.
6. Preheat oven to 390 F.
7. Season chicken breasts with salt and black pepper, and wrap 2 bacon slices around each chicken breast.

8 Arrange on a baking sheet that is lined with parchment paper, drizzle with oil and bake for 25-30 minutes until bacon is brown and crispy.

9 Serve with grilled fennel sprinkled with rosemary.

Per serving:

- Cal 487
- Fat 39g
- Net Carbs 5.2g
- Protein 27g

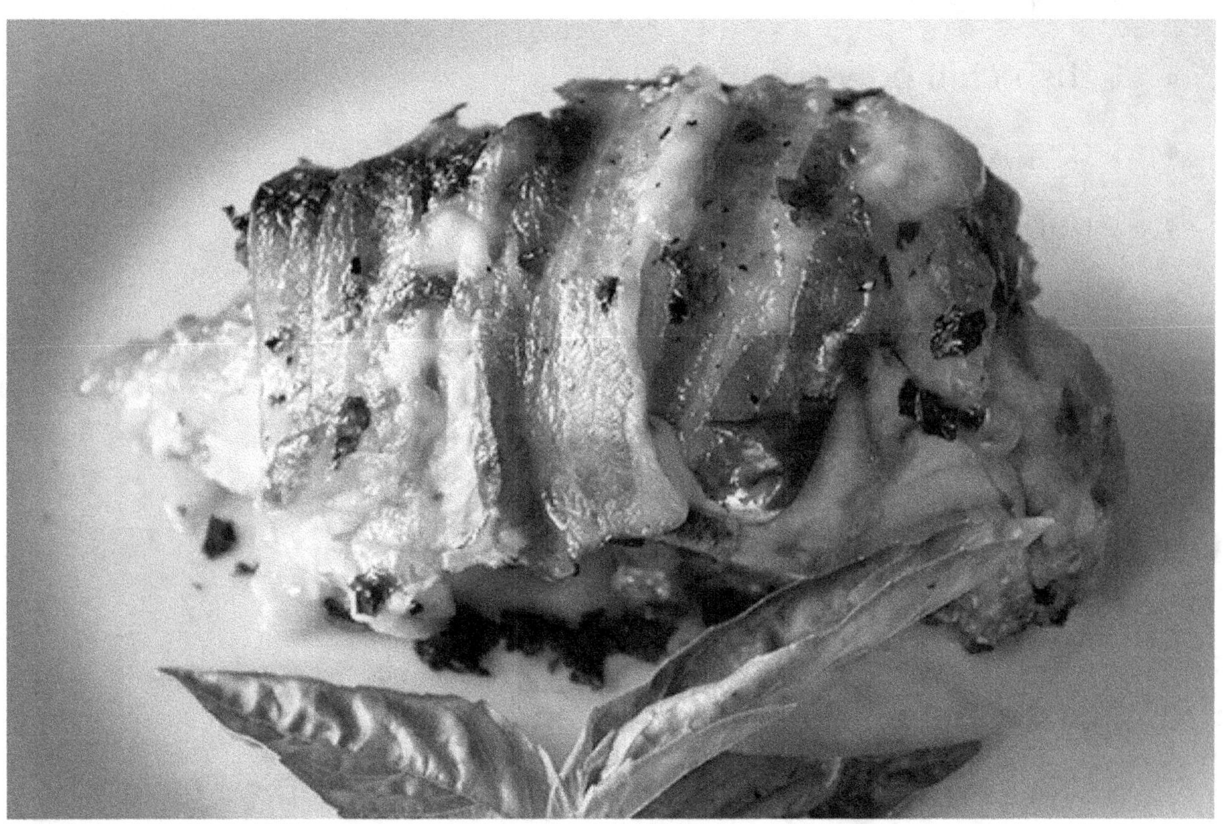

28. TOMATO & CHEESE CHICKEN CHILI

Ingredients

For 4 servings

- 1 tbsp butter
- 1 tbsp olive oil
- 1 lb chicken breasts, cubed
- ½ onion, chopped
- 1 cups tomatoes, chopped
- 2 oz tomato puree
- 1 tbsp chili powder
- 1 tbsp cumin
- 1 garlic clove, minced
- 1 habanero pepper, minced
- ½ cup mozzarella, shredded
- Salt and black pepper to taste

Directions

Total Time: approx. 40 minutes

1 Season the chicken with salt and black pepper.

2 Set a large pan over medium heat and add the chicken.

3 Cover with water and bring to a boil.

4 Cook until no longer pink, about 10 minutes.

5 Transfer the chicken to a flat surface to shred with forks; reserve the broth (about 2 cups).

6   In a pot, pour the butter and olive oil and set over medium heat.

7   Sauté onion and garlic until transparent, 3 minutes.

8   Stir in the chicken, tomatoes, cumin, habanero pepper, tomato puree, and chili powder for 1-2 minutes.

9   Adjust the seasoning and pour in the reserved broth; bring the mixture to a boil.

10 Reduce heat to simmer for about 10 minutes.

11 Top with mozzarella cheese and serve.

Per serving:

- Cal 322

- Fat 17g

- Net Carbs 6.2g

- Protein 29g

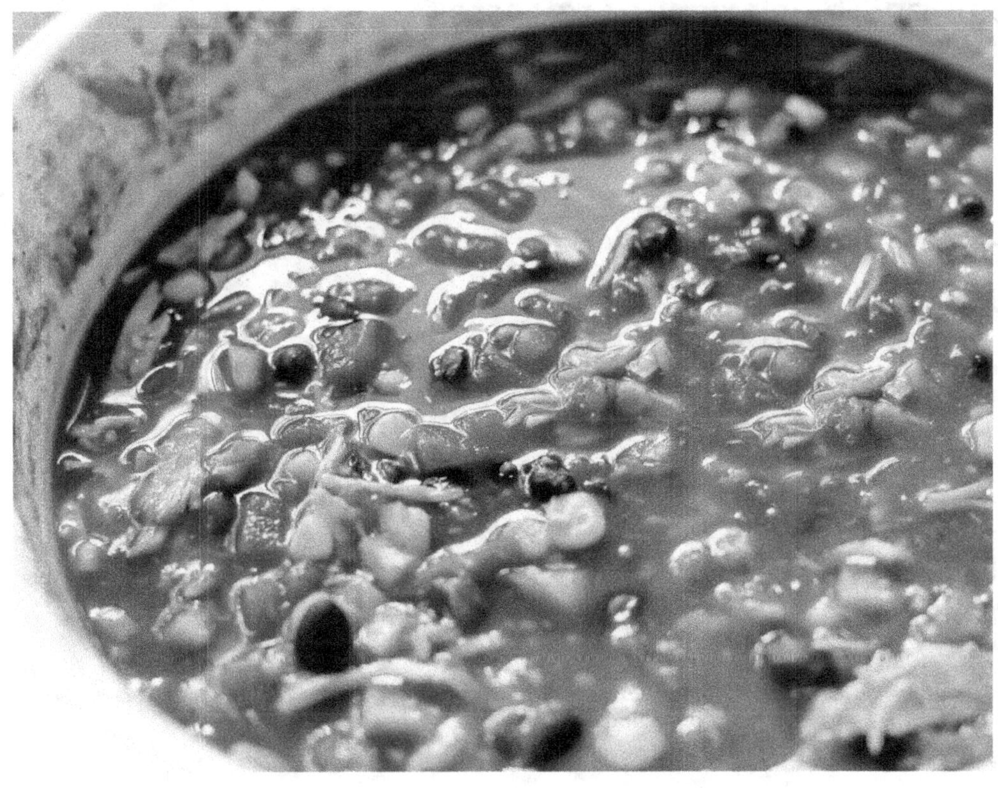

19. PAN-FRIED CHICKEN WITH ANCHOVY TAPENADE

Ingredients

For 2 servings

- 1 chicken breast, cut into 4 pieces
- 2 tbsp olive oil
- 1 garlic clove, minced

Tapenade

- 2 tbsp olive oil
- 1 cup black olives, pitted
- 1 oz anchovy fillets, rinsed
- 1 garlic clove, crushed
- Salt and black pepper to taste
- ¼ cup fresh basil, chopped
- 1 tbsp lemon juice

Directions

Total Time: approx. 20 minutes

1. Heat a pan over medium heat and add olive oil.

2. Stir in the garlic and cook for 2 minutes.

3. Place in the chicken pieces and cook each side for 4 minutes. Remove to a serving plate.

4. Chop the black olives and anchovy and put them in a food processor.

5. Add in olive oil, basil, lemon juice, salt, and black pepper, and blend well.

6. Spoon the tapenade over the chicken and serve.

Per serving:

- Cal 522

- Fat 37g

- Net Carbs 5.3g

- Protein 43g

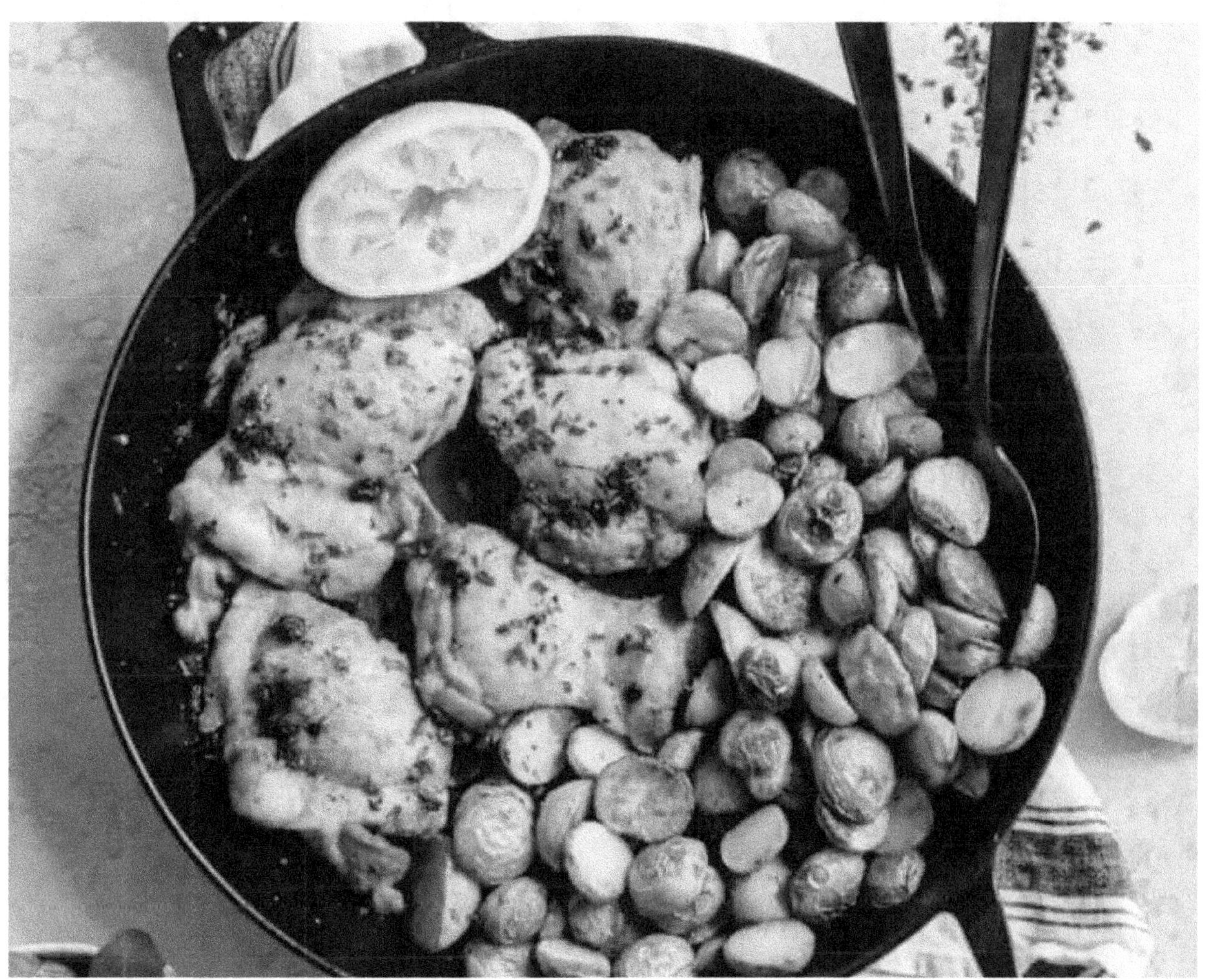

20. BAKED ZUCCHINI WITH CHICKEN AND CHEESE

Ingredients

For 4 servings

- 1 lb chicken breasts, cubed
- 1 tbsp butter
- 1 tbsp olive oil
- 1 red bell pepper, chopped
- 1 shallot, sliced
- 2 zucchinis, cubed
- 1 garlic clove, minced
- 1 tsp thyme
- Salt and black pepper to taste
- ½ cup cream cheese, softened
- ¼ cup mayonnaise
- 1 tbsp Worcestershire sauce
- 1 cup mozzarella, shredded

Directions

Total Time: approx. 45 minutes

1 Set oven to 370 F.

2 Heat the butter and olive oil in a pan over medium heat and add in the chicken.

3 Cook until lightly browned, about 5 minutes.

4 Place in shallot, zucchini cubes, black pepper, garlic, bell
   pepper, salt, and thyme.

5 Cook for 5 minutes until tender; set aside.

6 In a bowl, mix the cream cheese, mayonnaise, and
   Worcestershire sauce.

7 Stir in the chicken and sauteed vegetables.

8 Place the mixture into a greased baking dish and bake for
   20 minutes.

9 Sprinkle with mozzarella cheese and bake until browned,
   about 5 minutes.

Per serving:

- Cal 488

- Fat 38g

- Net Carbs 5.2g

- Protein 23g

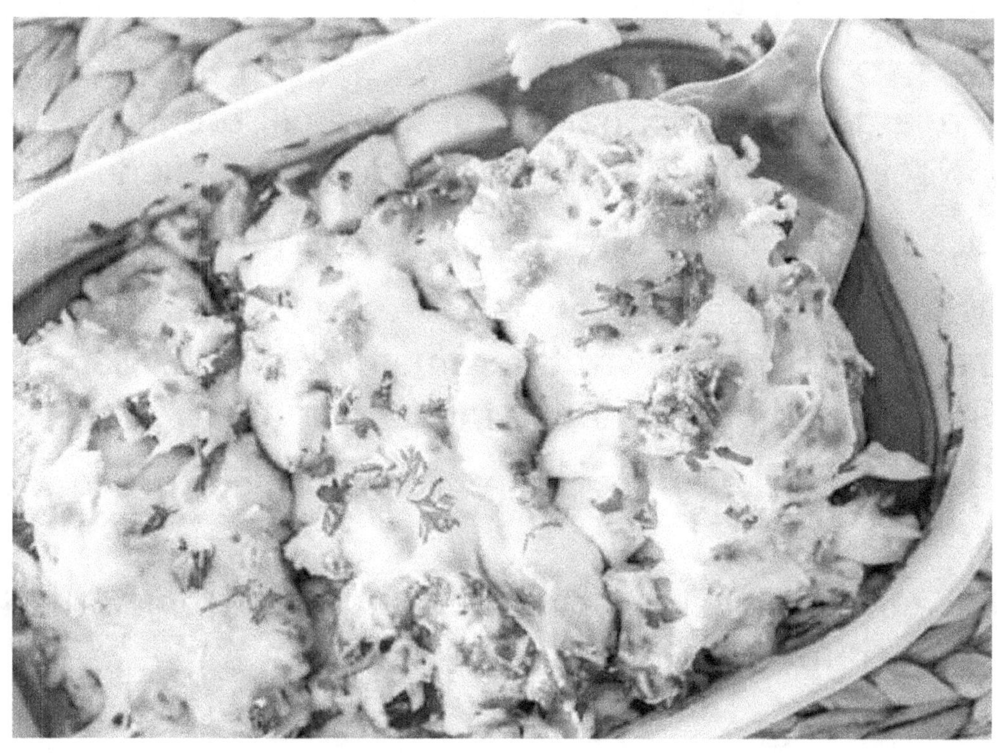

21. CHICKEN KABOBS WITH CELERY ROOT CHIPS

Ingredients

For 2 servings

- 4 tbsp olive oil
- 2 chicken breasts, cubed
- Salt and black pepper to taste
- 1 tsp dried oregano
- 1 tsp chili powder
- ¼ cup chicken broth
- 1 lb celery root, sliced

Directions

Total Time: approx. 60 minutes

1 Preheat oven to 400 F.

2 In a large bowl, mix half of the olive oil, oregano, chili powder, salt, black pepper and add the chicken.

3 Toss to coat and set in the fridge for 10 minutes.

4 Arrange the celery slices on a greased baking tray in an even layer, drizzle with the remaining olive oil, and sprinkle with salt and pepper. Bake for 10 minutes.

5 Take the chicken from the refrigerator and thread it onto skewers.

6 Place over the celery, pour in the chicken broth, then set in the oven for 30 minutes. Serve.

Per serving:

- Cal 365
- Fat 23g
- Net Carbs 4.6g
- Protein 35g

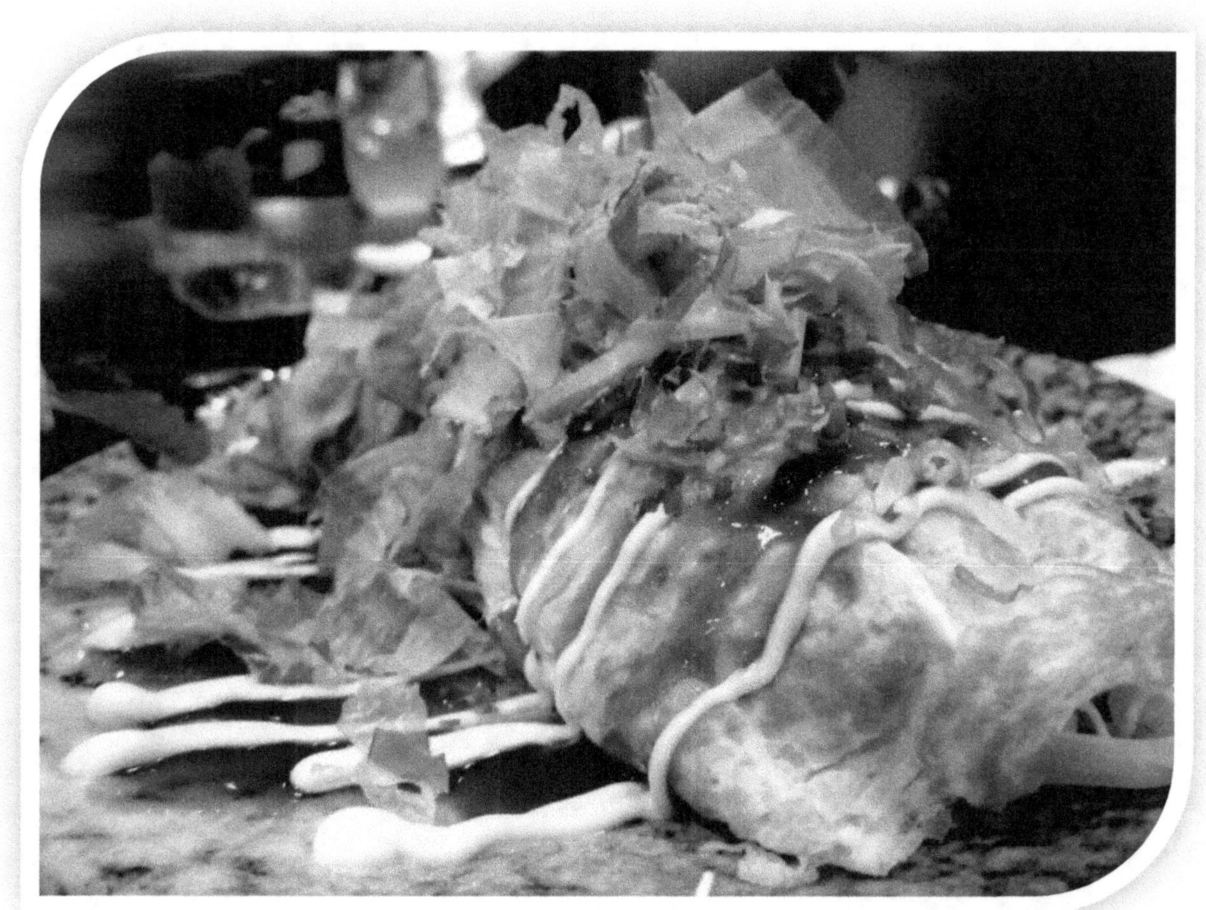

BEEF & LAMB

22. BEEF RAGOUT WITH PEPPER & GREEN BEANS

Ingredients

For 4 servings

- 1 lb chuck steak, trimmed and cubed
- 2 tbsp olive oil
- Salt and black pepper to taste
- 2 tbsp almond flour
- 4 green onions, diced
- ½ cup dry white wine
- 1 yellow bell pepper, diced
- 1 cup green beans, chopped
- 2 tsp Worcestershire sauce
- 4 oz tomato puree
- 3 tsp smoked paprika
- 1 cup beef broth
- Parsley leaves to garnish

Directions

Total Time: approx. 2 hours

1. Dredge the meat in the almond flour and set aside.
2. Place a large skillet over medium heat, add 1 tablespoon of oil to heat and then sauté the green onion, green beans, and bell pepper for 3 minutes.
3. Stir in the paprika and the remaining olive oil.

4 Add the beef and cook for 10 minutes while turning them halfway.

5 Stir in white wine, let it reduce by half, about 3 minutes, and add Worcestershire sauce, tomato puree, and beef broth.

6 Let the mixture boil for 2 minutes, then reduce the heat to lowest and let simmer for 1 ½ hours; stirring now and then.

7 Adjust the taste and dish the ragout.

8 Serve garnished with parsley.

Per serving:

- Cal 334
- Fat 22g
- Net Carbs 3.9g
- Protein 33g

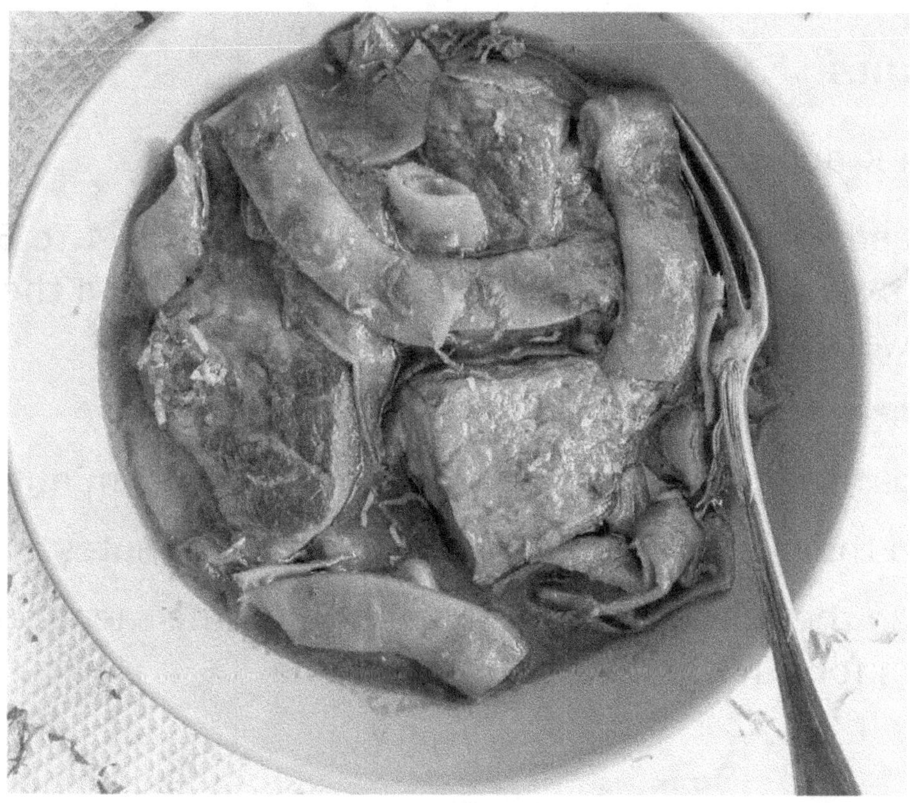

23. GRILLED BEEF ON SKEWERS WITH FRESH SALAD

Ingredients

For 2 servings

- 1 lb sirloin steak, boneless, cubed
- ¼ cup ranch dressing
- 1 red onion, sliced
- ½ tbsp white wine vinegar
- 1 tbsp extra virgin olive oil
- 2 ripe tomatoes, sliced
- 2 tbsp fresh parsley, chopped
- 1 cucumber, sliced
- Salt to taste

Directions

Total Time: approx. 20 minutes

1. Thread the beef cubes on the skewers, about 4 to 5 cubes per skewer. Brush half of the ranch dressing on the skewers (all around).
2. Preheat grill to high.
3. Place the skewers on the grill and cook for 6 minutes.
4. Turn the skewers and cook further for 6 minutes.
5. Brush the remaining ranch dressing on the meat and cook them for 1 more minute on each side.

6 In a salad bowl, mix together red onion, tomatoes, and cucumber, sprinkle with salt, vinegar, and extra virgin olive oil; toss to combine.

7 Top the salad with skewers and scatter the parsley all over.

Per serving:

- Cal 423
- Fat 24g
- Net Carbs 2.4g
- Protein 45g

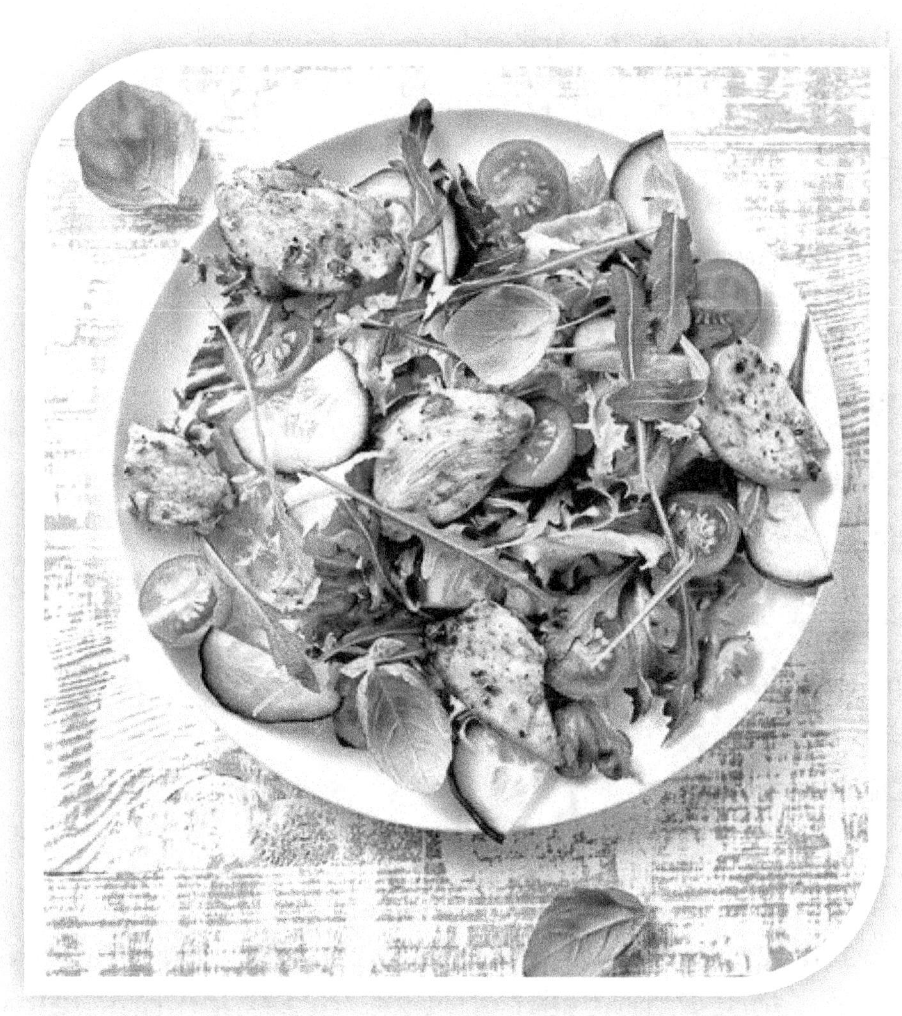

24. BEEF SAUSAGE & OKRA CASSEROLE

Ingredients

For 4 servings

- ½ cup marinara sauce, sugar- free
- 1 cup okra, trimmed
- 1 tbsp olive oil
- 1 celery stalk, chopped
- ¼ cup almond flour
- 1 egg
- 1 lb beef sausage, chopped
- Salt and black pepper to taste
- ½ tbsp dried parsley
- ¼ tsp red pepper flakes
- ¼ cup Parmesan cheese, grated
- 1 green onions, chopped
- ½ tsp garlic powder
- ¼ tsp dried oregano
- ½ cup ricotta cheese
- 1 cup cheddar cheese, grated

Directions

Total Time: approx. 35 minutes

1 In a bowl, combine the sausage, pepper, pepper flakes, oregano, egg, Parmesan cheese, green onions, almond flour, salt, parsley, celery, and garlic powder.

2   Form balls, lay them on a lined baking sheet, place in the
    oven at 390 F, and bake for 15 minutes.

3   Remove the balls from the oven and cover with half of the
    marinara sauce and okra.

4   Pour ricotta cheese all over, followed by the rest of the
    marinara sauce. Scatter the cheddar cheese and bake in
    the oven for 10 minutes.

5   Allow to cool before serving.

Per serving:

- Cal 479
- Fat 31g
- Net Carbs 4.3g
- Protein 39g

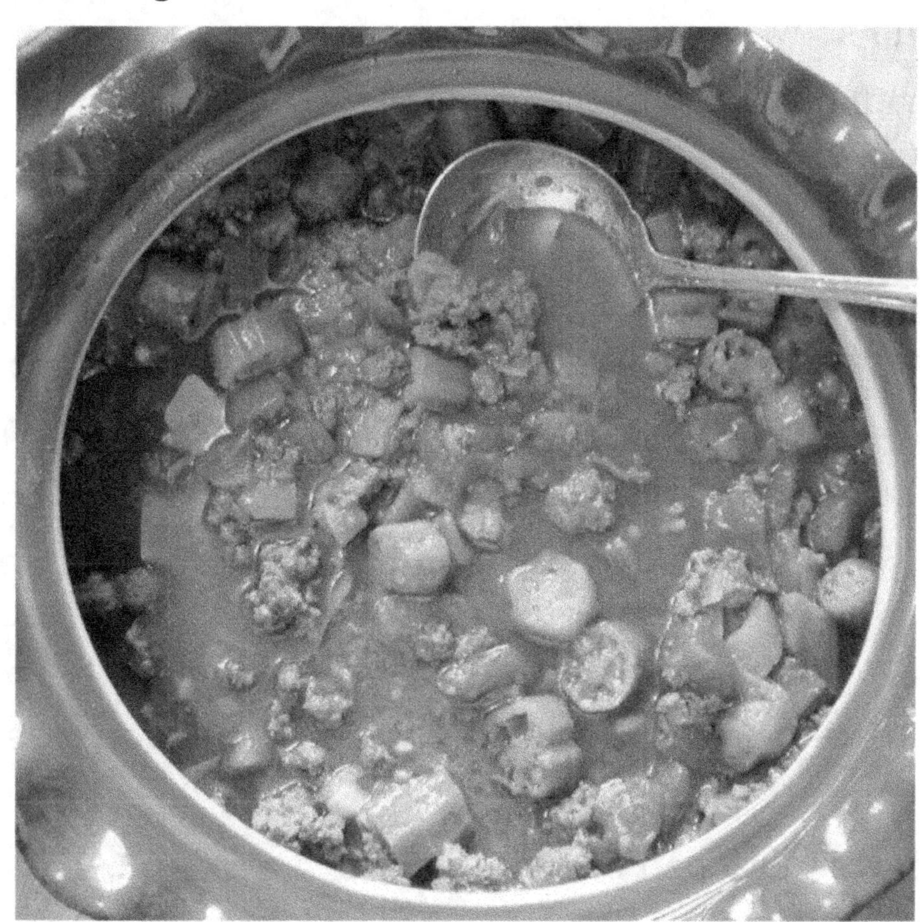

25. GRILLED BEEF STEAKS & VEGETABLE MEDLEY

Ingredients

For 2 servings

- 1 red bell pepper, seeded, cut into strips
- 2 sirloin beef steaks
- Salt and black pepper to taste
- 2 tbsp olive oil
- 1 ½ tbsp balsamic vinegar
- ¼ lb asparagus, trimmed
- ½ cup mushrooms, sliced
- ½ cup snow peas
- 1 small onion, quartered
- 1 garlic clove, sliced

Directions

Total Time: approx. 30 minutes

1 In a bowl, put asparagus, mushrooms, snow peas, bell pepper, onion, and garlic.

2 Mix salt, pepper, olive oil, and balsamic vinegar in a small bowl, and pour half of the mixture over the vegetables; stir to combine.

3 To the remaining oil mixture, add the beef and toss to coat well.

4 Preheat a grill pan over high heat.

5 Place the steaks in the grill pan and sear for 6-8 minutes on each side.

6 Remove the beef and set aside.

7 Pour the vegetables and marinade in the pan and cook for 5 minutes, turning once.

8 Share the vegetables into plates.

9 Top with beef and drizzle the sauce from the pan all and serve.

Per serving:

- Cal 488
- Fat 31g
- Net Carbs 4.1g
- Protein 57g

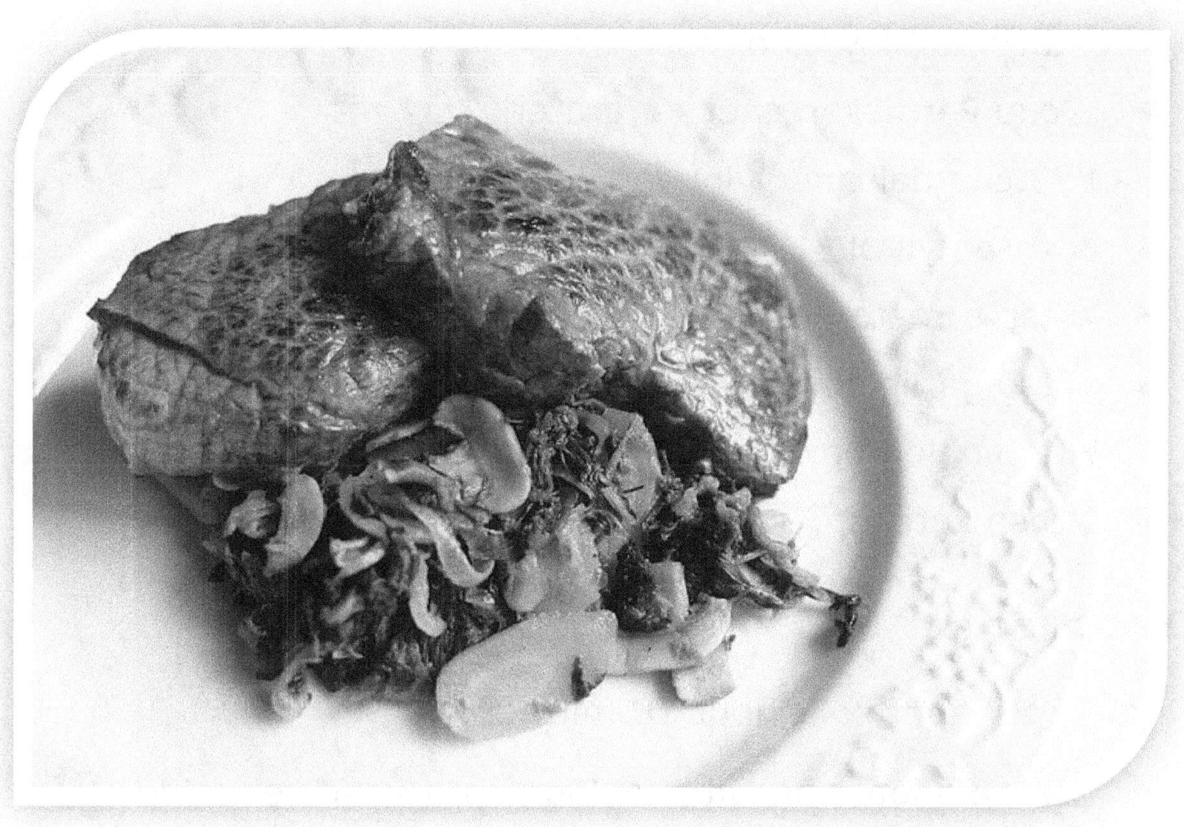

26. BEEF & MUSHROOM MEATLOAF

Ingredients

For 4 servings

Meatloaf

- 1 lb ground beef
- ½ onion, chopped
- 1 tbsp almond milk
- 1 tbsp almond flour
- 1 garlic clove, minced
- 1 cup sliced mushrooms
- 1 small egg
- Salt and black pepper to taste
- 1 tbsp parsley, chopped
- ⅓ cup Parmesan cheese, grated **Glaze**
- 1 /3 cup balsamic vinegar
- ¼ tbsp xylitol
- ¼ tsp tomato paste
- ¼ tsp garlic powder
- ¼ tsp onion powder
- 1 tbsp ketchup, sugar- free

Directions

Total Time: approx. 1 hour 10 minutes

1 Grease a loaf pan with cooking spray and set aside.

2 Preheat oven to 390 F.

3 Combine all meatloaf ingredients in a large bowl.

4 Press this mixture into the prepared loaf pan.

5 Bake in the oven for about 30 minutes.

6 To make the glaze, whisk all ingredients in a bowl.

7 Pour the glaze over the meatloaf.

8 Put the meatloaf back in the oven and cook for 20 more minutes.

9 Let meatloaf sit for 10 minutes before slicing.

10 Serve and enjoy!

Per serving:

- Cal 311
- Fat 21g
- Net Carbs 5.5g
- Protein 24g

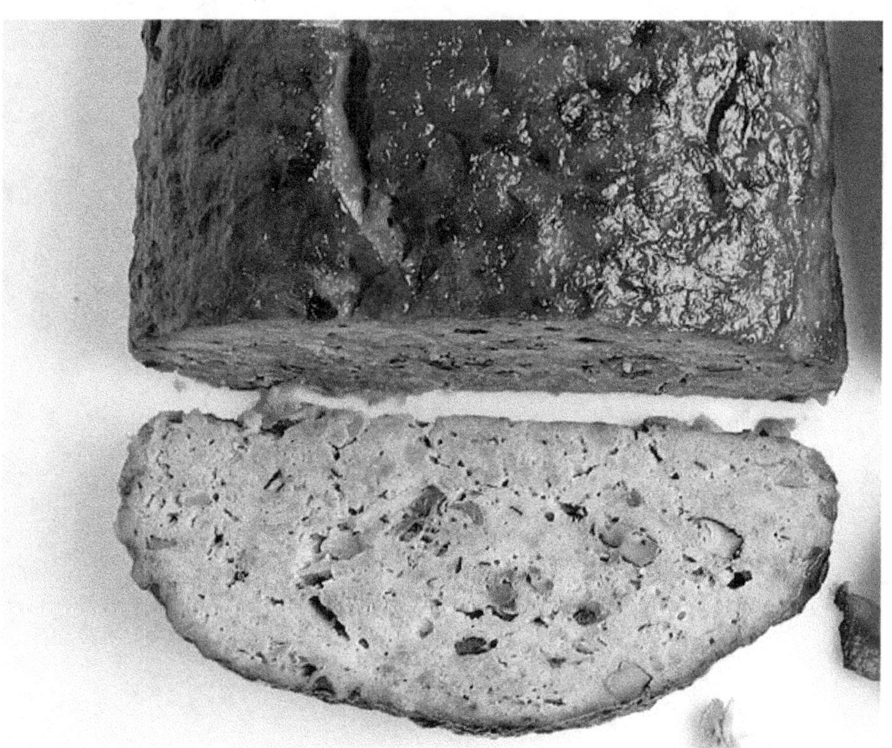

FISH & SEAFOOD

27. MEDITERRANEAN TILAPIA BAKE

Ingredients

For 2 servings

- 2 tilapia fillets
- 2 garlic cloves, minced
- 1 cup canned tomatoes
- ¼ tbsp chili powder
- 2 tbsp white wine
- 1 tbsp olive oil
- ½ red onion, chopped
- 1 tbsp parsley, chopped
- 1 tsp basil, chopped
- 1 black olives, halved

Directions

Total Time: approx. 30 minutes

1 Preheat oven to 350 F.
2 Heat the olive oil in a skillet over medium heat and stir-fry the onion and garlic for about 3 minutes.
3 Stir in tomatoes, olives, chili powder, and wine and bring the mixture to a boil.
4 Reduce the heat and simmer for 5 minutes.
5 Put the tilapia in a baking dish, pour over the sauce and bake for 12-15 minutes.
6 Serve garnished with basil and parsley.

Per serving:

- Cal 282
- Fat 15g
- Net Carbs 6g
- Protein 23g

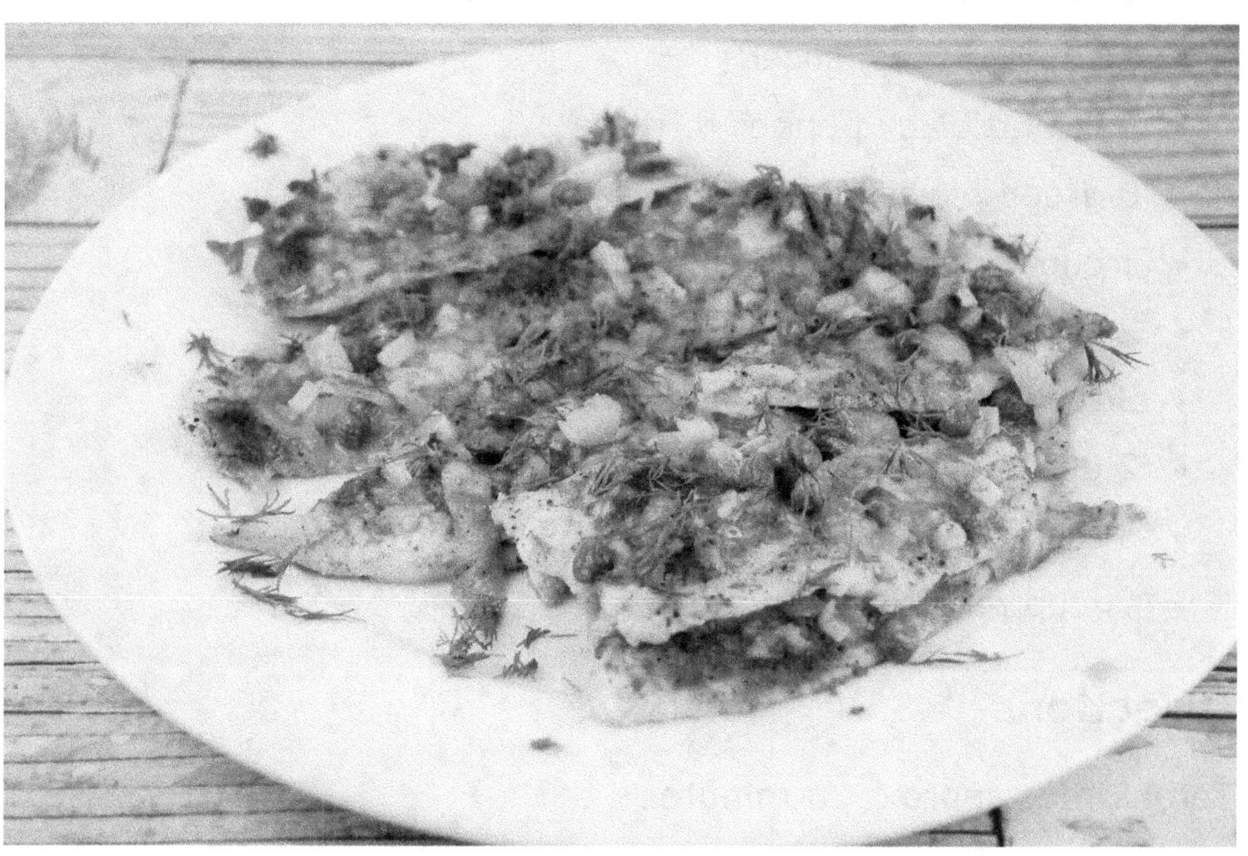

28. GRILLED SALMON WITH RADISH SALAD

Ingredients

For 4 servings

- 1 lb skinned salmon, cut into 4 steaks each
- 1 cup radishes, sliced
- Salt and black pepper to taste
- 8 green olives, chopped
- 1 cup arugula
- 2 large tomatoes, diced
- 3 tbsp red wine vinegar
- 2 green onions, sliced
- 3 tbsp olive oil
- ¼ cup parsley, chopped

Directions

Total Time: approx. 20 minutes

1. In a bowl, mix the radishes, olives, arugula, tomatoes, vinegar, green onion, 2 tbsp of olive oil, and parsley.
2. Put in the fridge while preparing the salmon.
3. Preheat your grill to high.
4. Season the salmon steaks with salt and pepper and drizzle with the remaining olive oil.
5. Grill the salmon on both sides for 8 minutes in total.
6. Serve warm with the radish salad.

Per serving:

- Cal 338
- Fat 22g
- Net Carbs 3.1g
- Protein 28g

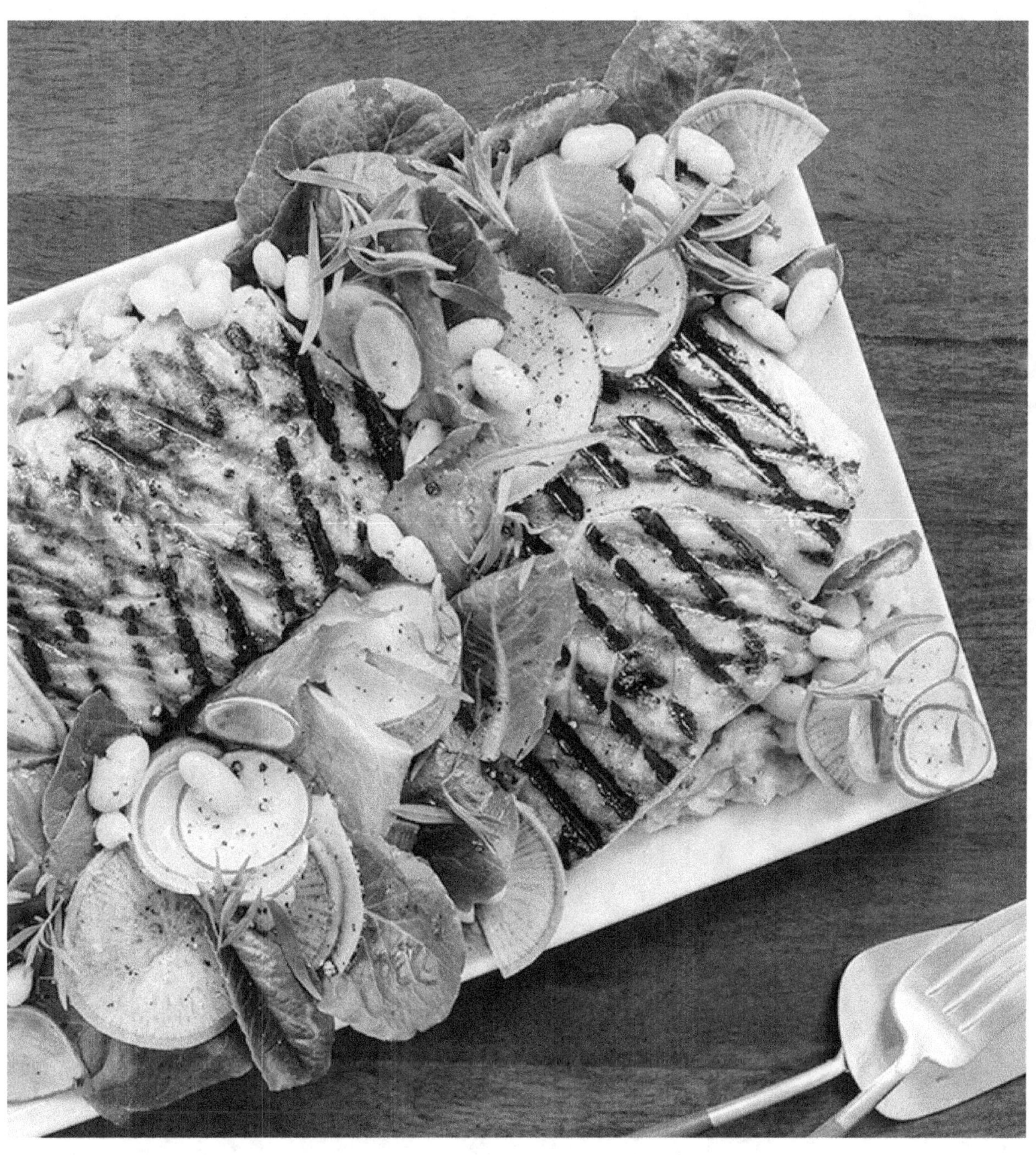

VEGETABLE SIDES & DAIRY

29. CHEDDAR STUFFED ZUCCHINI

Ingredients

For 2 servings

- 4 tbsp butter
- 1 zucchini, halved
- 1 ½ oz baby kale
- 2 garlic cloves, minced
- 2 tbsp tomato sauce
- 1 cup cheddar cheese
- Salt and black pepper to taste

Directions

Total Time: approx. 40 minutes

1. Preheat oven to 375 F.
2. Scoop out zucchini pulp with a spoon.
3. Keep the flesh.
4. Grease a baking sheet with cooking spray and place in the zucchini boats.
5. Melt butter in a skillet over medium heat and sauté garlic until fragrant and slightly browned, 4 minutes.
6. Add in kale and zucchini pulp.
7. Cook until the kale wilts; season with salt and pepper.
8. Spoon tomato sauce into the boats and spread to coat evenly.
9. Top with kale mixture and sprinkle with cheddar cheese.

10 Bake for 25 minutes.

Per serving:

- Cal 617
- Net Carbs 4g
- Fat 61g
- Protein 19g

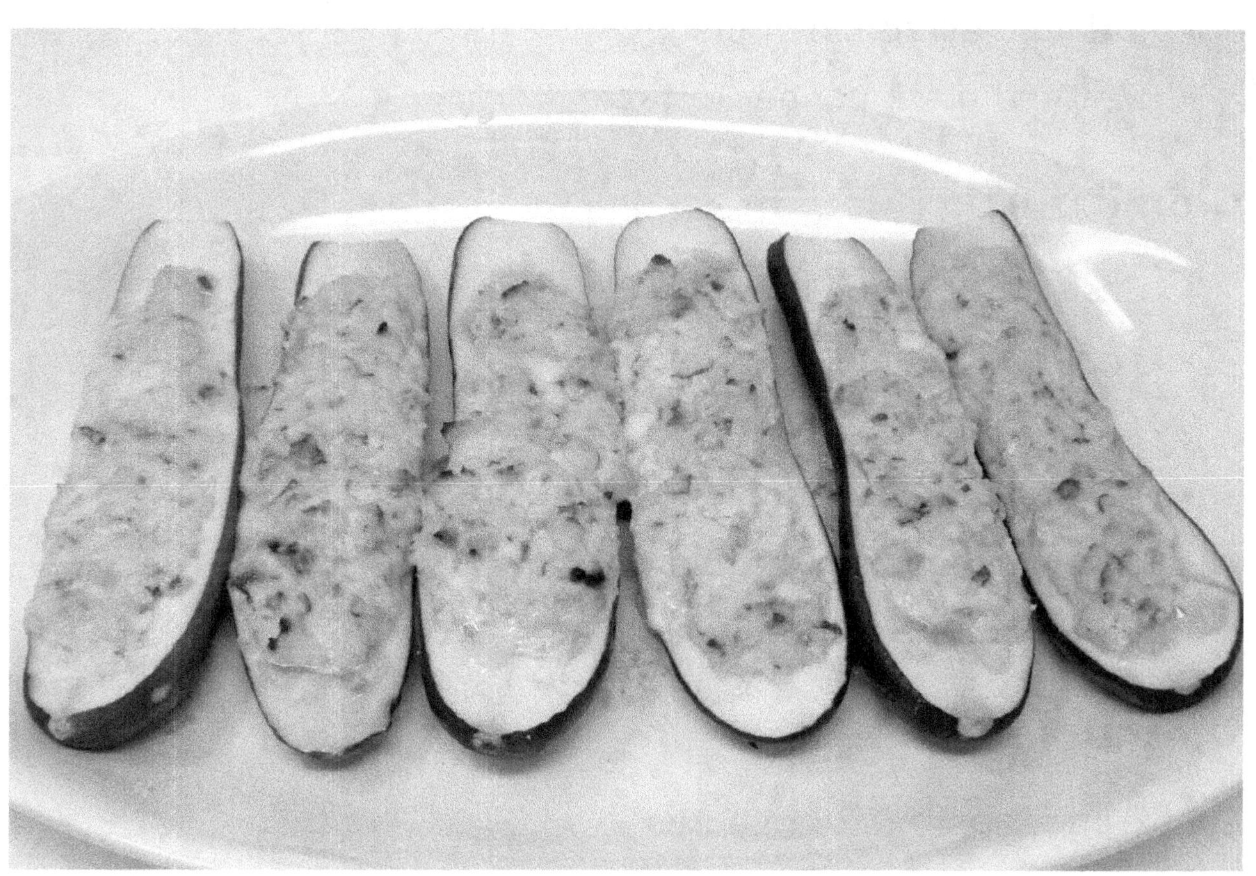

30. BUTTERNUT SQUASH ROAST WITH CHIMICHURRI

Ingredients

For 4 servings

- 1 lb butternut squash
- 1 tbsp butter, melted
- 3 tbsp toasted pine nuts
- Salt and black pepper to taste

Chimichurri:

- Zest and juice of 1 lemon
- 1 jalapeño pepper, chopped
- 1 cup olive oil
- 2 garlic cloves, minced
- ½ cup chopped fresh parsley
- ½ red bell pepper, chopped

Directions

Total Time: approx. 25 minutes

1 Add all the chimichurri ingredients to a food processor and grind until desired consistency is achieved; adjust the seasoning. Keep in the fridge until ready to use.

2 Slice the squash into rounds and remove the seeds.

3 Drizzle with butter and season with salt and pepper.

4 Preheat a grill pan over medium heat and cook the squash for 5-6 minutes on each side.

5 Scatter pine nuts on top and serve with chimichurri.

Per serving:

- Cal 647
- Net Carbs 6g
- Fat 44g
- Protein 49g

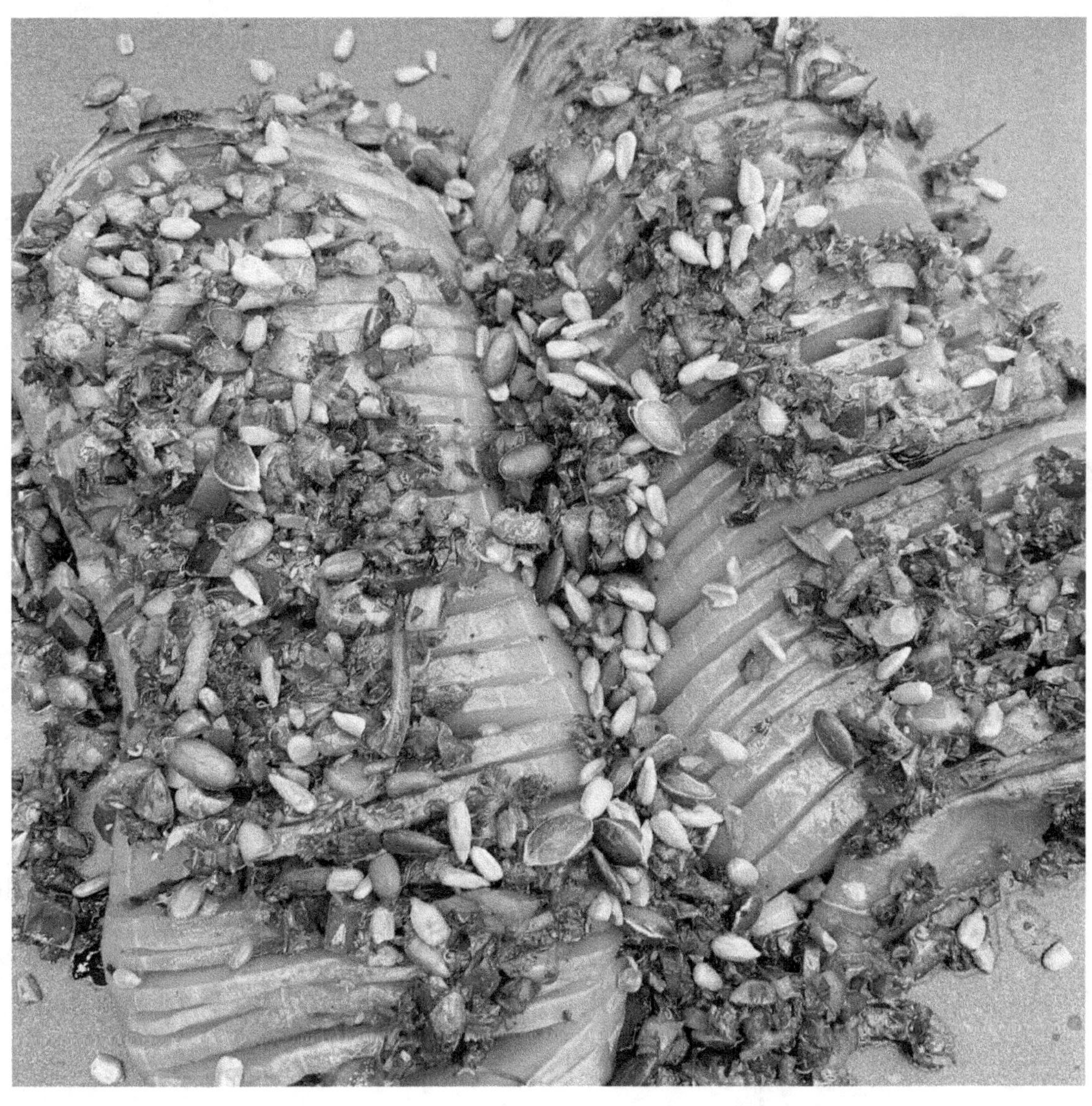

31. ROASTED PEPPER WITH TOFU

Ingredients

For 4 servings

- 2 ½ cups cubed tofu
- 4 orange bell peppers
- 1 cucumber, diced
- 1 large tomato, chopped
- 3 oz cream cheese
- ¾ cup mayonnaise
- 1 tbsp melted butter
- 1 tsp dried parsley
- 1 tsp dried basil
- Salt and black pepper to taste

Directions

Total Time: approx. 25 minutes

1 Preheat a broiler to 450 F.

2 Line a baking sheet with parchment paper.

3 In a salad bowl, combine cream cheese, mayonnaise, cucumber, tomato, salt, pepper, and parsley; refrigerate.

4 Arrange bell peppers and tofu on the baking sheet, drizzle with melted butter, and season with basil, salt, and pepper.

5 Bake for 15 minutes until the peppers have charred lightly and the tofu browned.

6 Serve with chilled salad and enjoy!

Per serving:

- Cal 838
- Net Carbs 8g
- Fat 81g
- Protein 31g

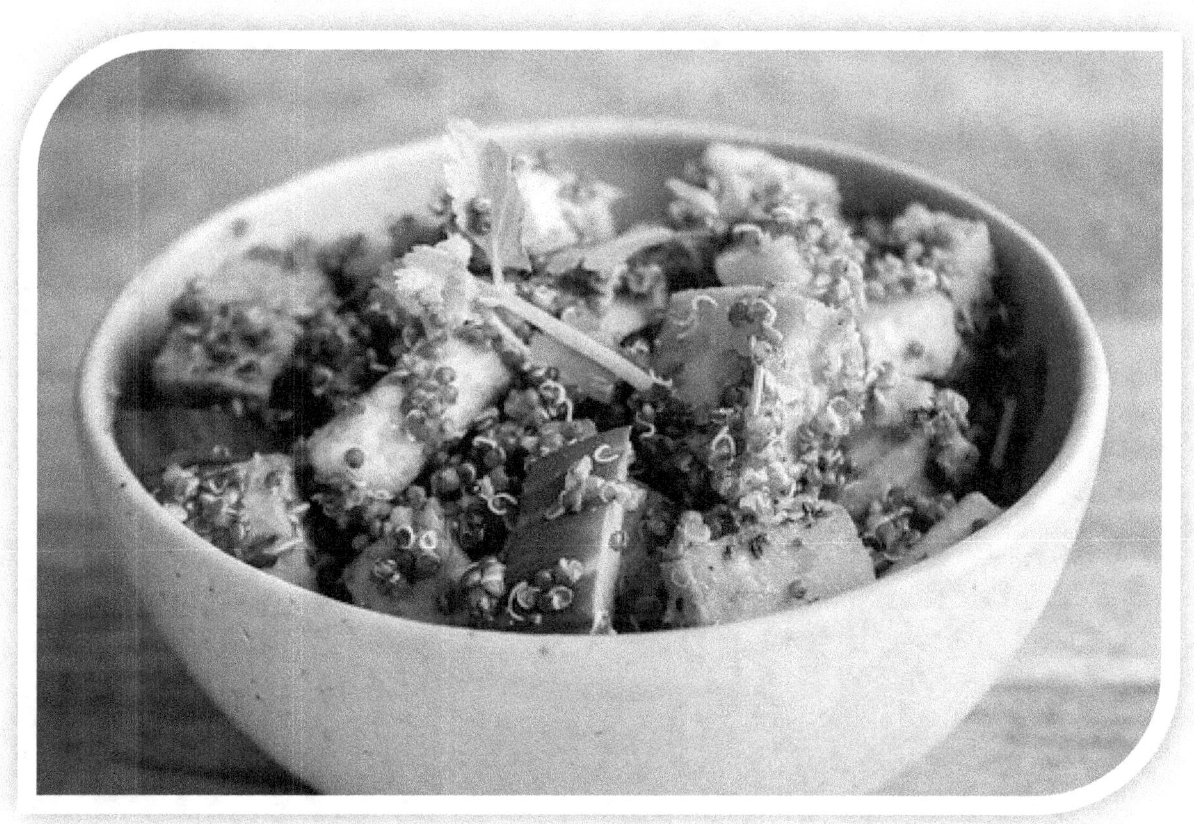

VEGAN

32. TOFU & VEGETABLE STIR-FRY

Ingredients

For 2 servings

- 2 tbsp olive oil
- 1 ½ cups tofu, cubed
- 1 ½ tbsp flaxseed meal
- Salt and black pepper to taste
- 1 garlic clove, minced
- 1 tbsp soy sauce, sugar- free
- ½ head broccoli, cut into florets
- 1 tsp onion powder
- 1 cup mushrooms, sliced
- 1 tbsp sesame seeds

Directions

Total Time: approx. 15 min + chilling time

1 In a bowl, add onion powder, tofu, salt, soy sauce, black pepper, flaxseed, and garlic.

2 Toss the mixture to coat and allow to marinate in the fridge for 20-30 minutes.

3 In a pan, warm the olive oil over medium heat.

4 Add the broccoli, mushrooms, and tofu mixture and stir-fry for 6-8 minutes.

5 Serve sprinkled with sesame seeds.

Per serving:

- Cal 423
- Fat 31g
- Net Carbs 7.3g
- Protein 25g

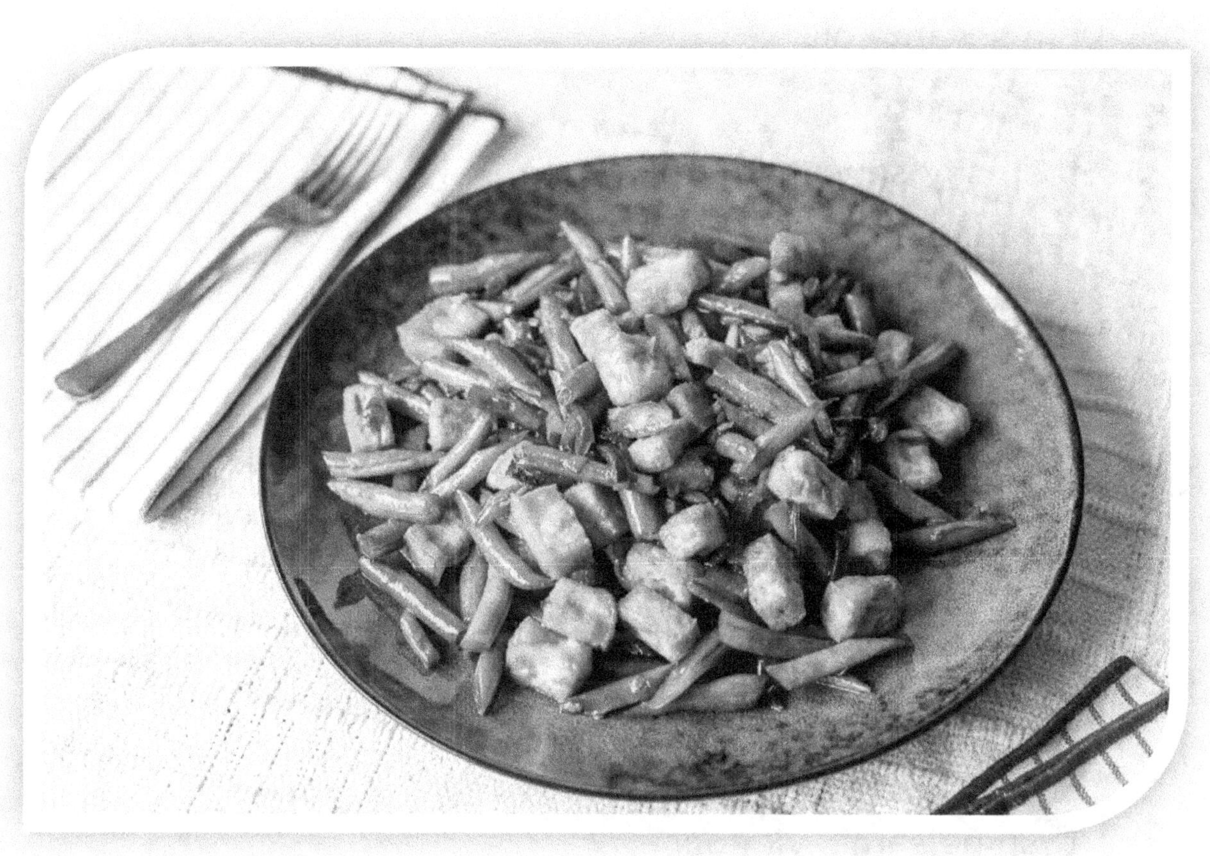

33. GRILLED TOFU KABOBS WITH ARUGULA SALAD

Ingredients

For 4 servings

- 14 oz firm tofu, cut into strips
- 4 tsp sesame oil
- 1 lemon, juiced
- 5 tbsp soy sauce, sugar- free
- 3 tsp garlic powder
- 3 tbsp coconut flour
- 4 ½ cup sesame seeds

Arugula salad

- 4 cups arugula, chopped
- 2 tsp extra virgin olive oil
- 2 tbsp pine nuts
- Salt and black pepper to taste
- 1 tbsp balsamic vinegar

Directions

Total Time: approx. 30 min + chilling time

1 Stick the tofu strips on the skewers, height-wise, and place them onto a plate.

2 In a bowl, mix sesame oil, lemon juice, soy sauce, garlic powder, and coconut flour.

3 Pour the soy sauce mixture over the tofu and turn in the sauce to coat.

4 Cover the dish and place in the fridge for 2 hours.

5 Heat the griddle pan over high heat.

6 Rool the tofu in the sesame seeds and grill until golden brown on both sides, about 12 minutes in total.

7 Arrange the arugula on a serving plate.

8 Drizzle over olive oil and balsamic vinegar and season with salt and black pepper.

9 Sprinkle with pine nuts and place the tofu kabobs on top to serve.

Per serving:

- Cal 411
- Fat 33g
- Net Carbs 7.1g
- Protein 22g

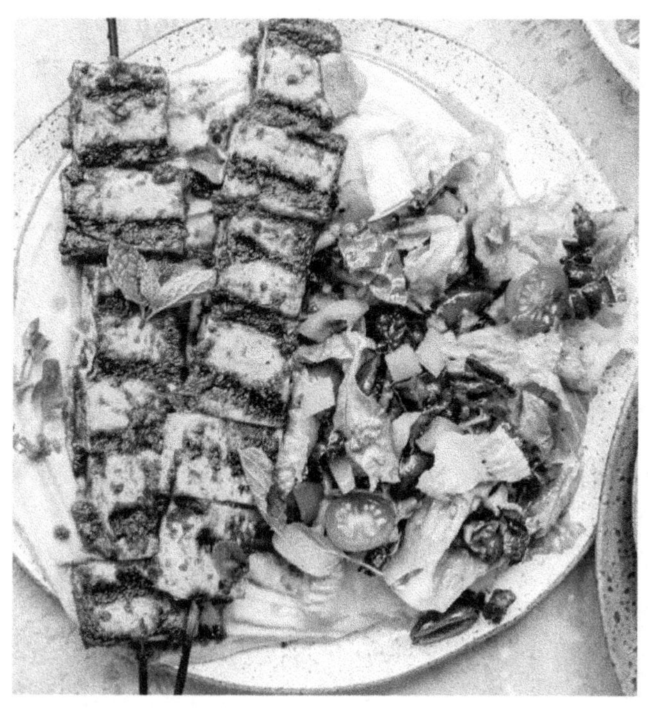

SNACKS & APPETIZERS

34. CHEESE & NUT ZUCCHINI BOATS

Ingredients

For 4 servings

- 2 medium zucchinis, halved
- 1 cup cauliflower rice
- 2 tbsp olive oil
- ¼ cup vegetable broth
- 1 ¼ cup diced tomatoes
- 1 red onion, chopped
- ¼ cup pine nuts
- ¼ cup hazelnuts
- 1 tbsp balsamic vinegar
- 1 tbsp smoked paprika
- 1 cup grated Monterey Jack
- 4 tbsp chopped cilantro

Directions

Total Time: approx. 35 minutes

1 Preheat oven to 350 F.
2 Pour cauli rice and broth in a pot and cook for 5 minutes.
3 Fluff the cauli rice and allow cooling.
4 Scoop the flesh out of the zucchini halves and chop the pulp. Brush the zucchini shells with some olive oil.
5 In a bowl, mix cauli rice, tomatoes, red onion, pine nuts, hazelnuts, cilantro, vinegar, paprika, and zucchini pulp.

Spoon the mixture into the zucchini halves, drizzle with remaining olive oil, and sprinkle the cheese on top.

6 Bake for 20 minutes until the cheese melts.

7 Serve.

Per serving:

- Cal 328
- Net Carbs 4.9g
- Fat 31g
- Protein 12g

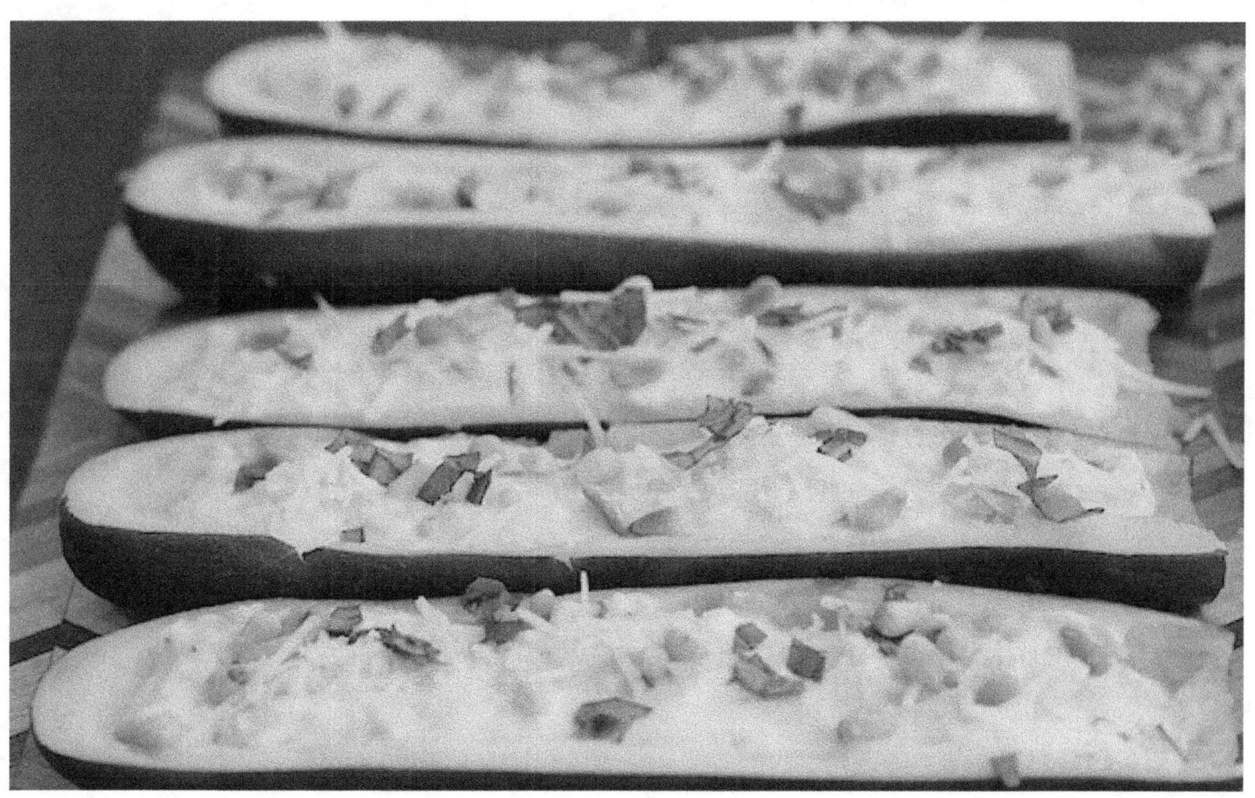

35. BAKED EGGPLANT CHIPS WITH SALAD & AIOLI

Ingredients

For 4 servings

- 2 eggplants, sliced
- 1 egg, beaten
- 3 ½ oz cooked beets, shredded
- 3 ½ oz red cabbage, shredded
- 2 cups almond flour
- 2 tbsp butter, melted
- 2 egg yolks
- 2 garlic cloves, minced
- 1 cup olive oil
- ½ tsp red chili flakes
- 1 tbsp lemon juice
- 2 tbsp yogurt
- 2 tbsp fresh cilantro, chopped
- Salt and black pepper to taste

Directions

Total Time: approx. 30 minutes

1　Preheat oven to 400 F.

2　On a deep plate, mix flour, salt, and pepper.

3 Dip eggplants into the egg, then in the flour.

4 Place on a greased baking sheet and brush with butter.

5 Bake for 15 minutes.

6 To make aioli, whisk egg yolks with garlic.

7 Gradually pour in ¾ cup olive oil while whisking.

8 Stir in chili flakes, salt, pepper, 1 tbsp of lemon juice, and yogurt.

9 In a salad bowl, mix beets, cabbage, cilantro, remaining oil, remaining lemon juice, salt, and pepper; toss to coat.

10 Serve the fries with the aioli and beet salad.

Per serving:

- Cal 847

- Net Carbs 8g

- Fat 81g

- Protein 26g

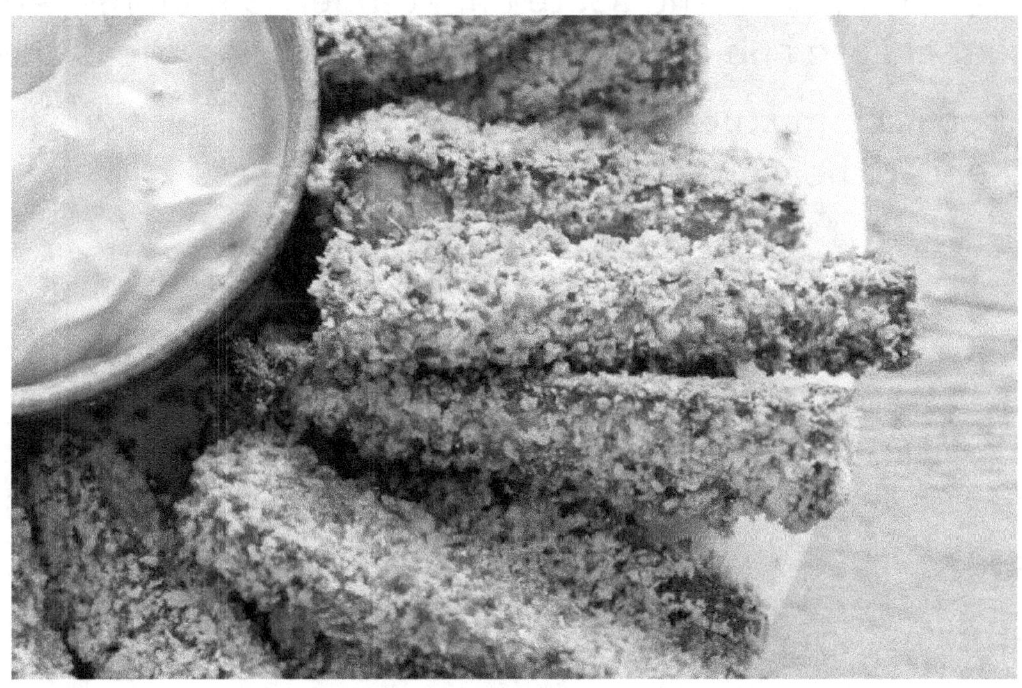

36. MUSHROOM & CHEESE LETTUCE WRAPS

Ingredients

For 4 servings

- 1 iceberg lettuce, leaves extracted
- 4 oz baby Bella mushrooms, sliced
- 1 cup grated cheddar cheese
- 2 tbsp butter
- 1 lb goat cheese, crumbled
- 1 large tomato, sliced

Directions

Total Time: approx. 20 minutes

1. Warm butter in a skillet over medium heat.
2. Add mushrooms and sauté until tender, 6 minutes. Add in goat cheese and cook for 5 minutes, stirring occasionally.
3. Spoon the mixture into the lettuce leaves, sprinkle with cheddar cheese, and top with tomato slices.
4. Serve.

Per serving:

- Cal 617
- Net Carbs 3g
- Fat 52g
- Protein 32g

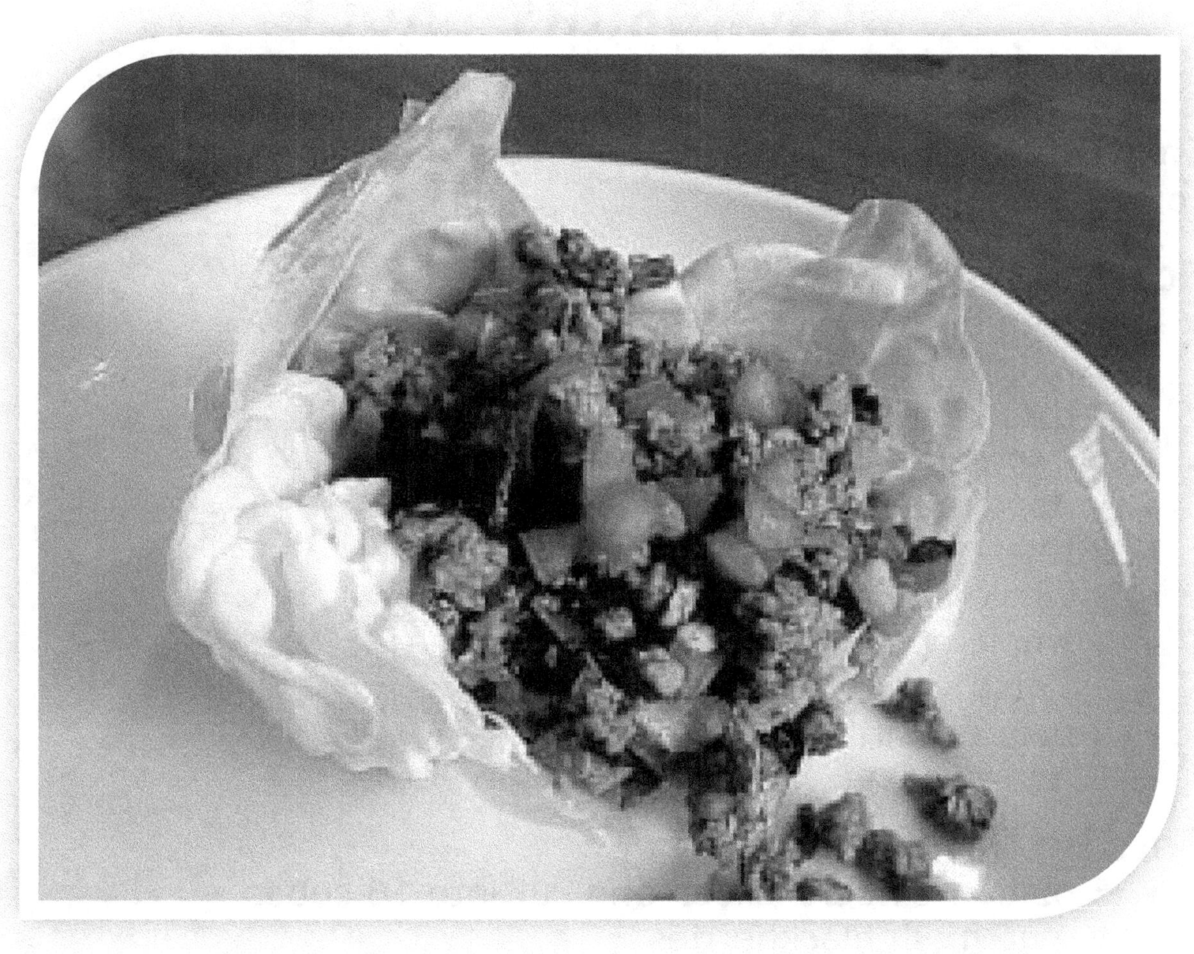

37. CAMEMBERT BITES WITH BLACKBERRY SAUCE

Ingredients

For 4 servings

For the pastry cups

- ¼ cup butter, cold and crumbled
- ¼ cup almond flour
- 3 tbsp coconut flour
- ½ tsp xanthan gum
- ¼ tsp cream of tartar
- 3 tbsp cream cheese, softened
- 3 whole eggs, unbeaten
- 1 whole egg, beaten
- 1 ½ tsp vanilla extract
- 3 tbsp erythritol
- ½ tsp salt

For the filling

- 5 oz Camembert, sliced and cut into 16 cubes
- ½ cup fresh blackberries
- 1 tsp butter
- 1 yellow onion, chopped
- 3 tbsp red wine
- 1 tbsp balsamic vinegar
- 5 tbsp erythritol

Directions

Total Time: approx. 40 min + chilling time

1. Preheat oven to 360 F.
2. Turn a muffin tray upside down and lightly grease with cooking spray.
3. In a bowl, mix almond and coconut flours, xanthan gum, and salt.
4. Add in cream cheese, cream of tartar, and butter and mix until crumbly.
5. Stir in erythritol and vanilla extract until mixed.

6   Then, pour in three eggs, one after another, while mixing until formed into a ball.
7   Flatten the dough on a clean flat surface, cover with plastic wrap, and refrigerate for 1 hour.
8   Dust a clean flat surface with almond flour, unwrap the dough, and roll out the dough into a large rectangle.
9   Cut into 16 squares and press each onto each muffin mound on the tray to form a bowl shape.
10 Brush with the beaten egg and bake for 10 minutes.
11 To make the filling, melt butter in a skillet and sauté onion for 3 minutes.
12 Stir in red wine, balsamic vinegar, erythritol, and blackberries.
13 Cook until the berries become jammy and wine reduces, 10 minutes.
14 Set aside. Take out the tray and place cheese cubes in each pastry.
15 Return to oven and bake for 3 minutes.
16 Spoon a tsp each of the blackberry sauce on top.
17 Serve and enjoy!

Per serving:
- Cal 369
- Net Carbs 4.4g
- Fat 32g
- Protein 14g

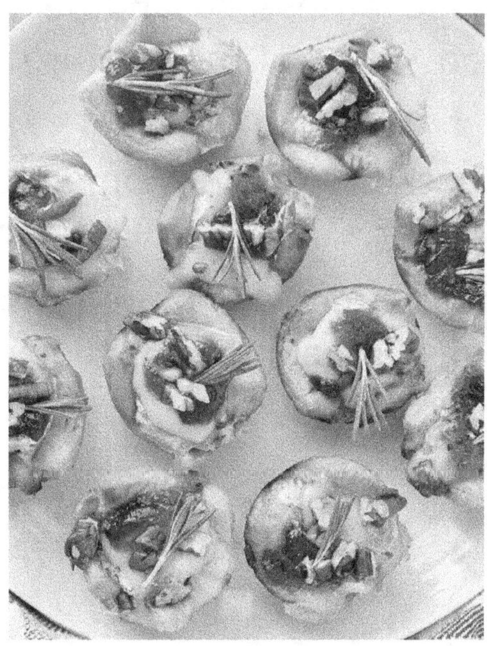

38. BASIL SPINACH & ZUCCHINI LASAGNA

Ingredients

For 4 servings

- 2 zucchinis, sliced
- Salt and black pepper to taste
- 2 cups feta cheese
- 2 cups mozzarella, shredded
- 3 cups tomato sauce
- 1 cup spinach
- 1 tbsp basil, chopped

Directions

Total Time: approx. 50 minutes

1 Preheat oven to 370 F.

2 Mix feta, mozzarella cheese, salt, and pepper to evenly combine and spread ¼ cup of the mixture at the bottom of a greased baking dish.

3 Layer 1/3 of the zucchini slices on top, spread 1 cup of tomato sauce over, and scatter a 1/3 cup of spinach on top.

4 Repeat the layering process two more times to exhaust the ingredients while finally making sure to layer with the last ¼ cup of cheese mixture.

5 Bake for 35 minutes until the cheese has a nice golden brown color.

6 Remove the dish, sit for 5 minutes and serve sprinkled with
   basil.

Per serving:

- Cal 411
- Fat 43g
- Net Carbs 3.2g
- Protein 6.5g

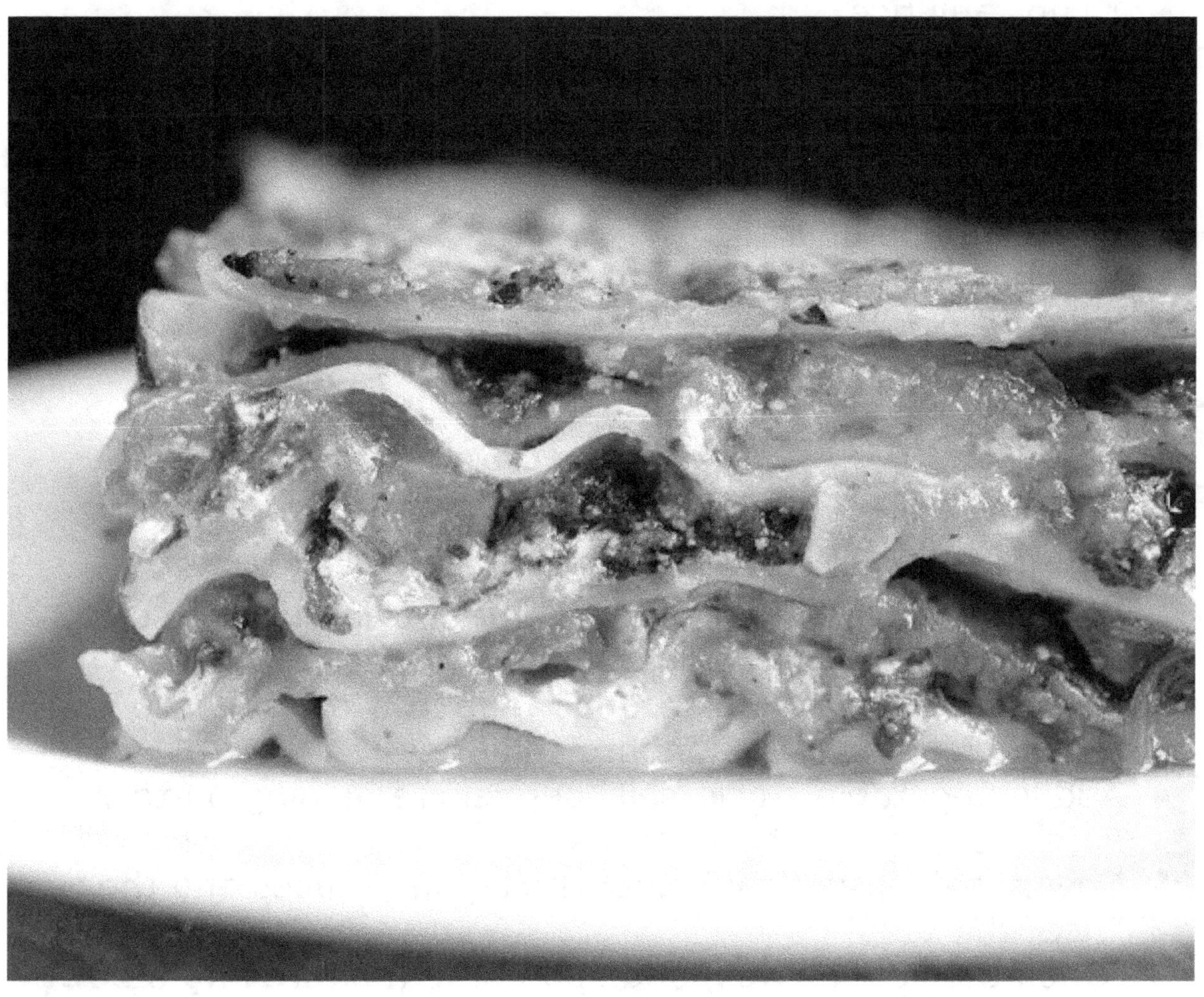

39. CAULI RICE ARANCINI

Ingredients

For 4 servings

- 2 tbsp butter
- 2 tbsp olive oil
- 2 eggs
- 1 white onion, finely chopped
- 2 scallions, chopped
- 2 garlic cloves, minced
- 1 cup cauli rice
- ¼ cup white wine
- ¼ cup vegetable stock
- ¼ cup grated Parmesan
- ½ cup ricotta cheese
- 1 cup almond flour
- ½ cup golden flaxseed meal
- Salt and black pepper to taste

Directions

Total Time: approx. 30 minutes

1 Heat butter in a saucepan over medium heat.
2 Stir in garlic and onion and cook until fragrant and soft, 3 minutes.
3 Mix in cauli rice for 30 seconds; add in wine, stir, allow reduction and absorption into cauli rice.
4 Add in vegetable stock, salt, pepper, remaining butter, Parmesan and ricotta cheeses.
5 Cover the pot and cook until the liquid reduces and the "rice" thickens.
6 Open the lid, stir well, and spoon the mixture into a bowl to cool.
7 Mold the dough into mini patties, 14-16 pieces; set aside.
8 Heat olive oil in a skillet over medium heat.

9 Pour the almond flour onto a plate, the golden flaxseed
   meal in another, and beat the eggs in a medium bowl.
10 Lightly dredge each patty in the flour, then in eggs, and
   then coat them in the flaxseed meal.
11 Fry in the oil until compacted and golden brown, 2 minutes
   per side. Garnish with scallions and serve.

Per serving:

- Cal 359
- Net Carbs 6.2g
- Fat 29g
- Protein 13g

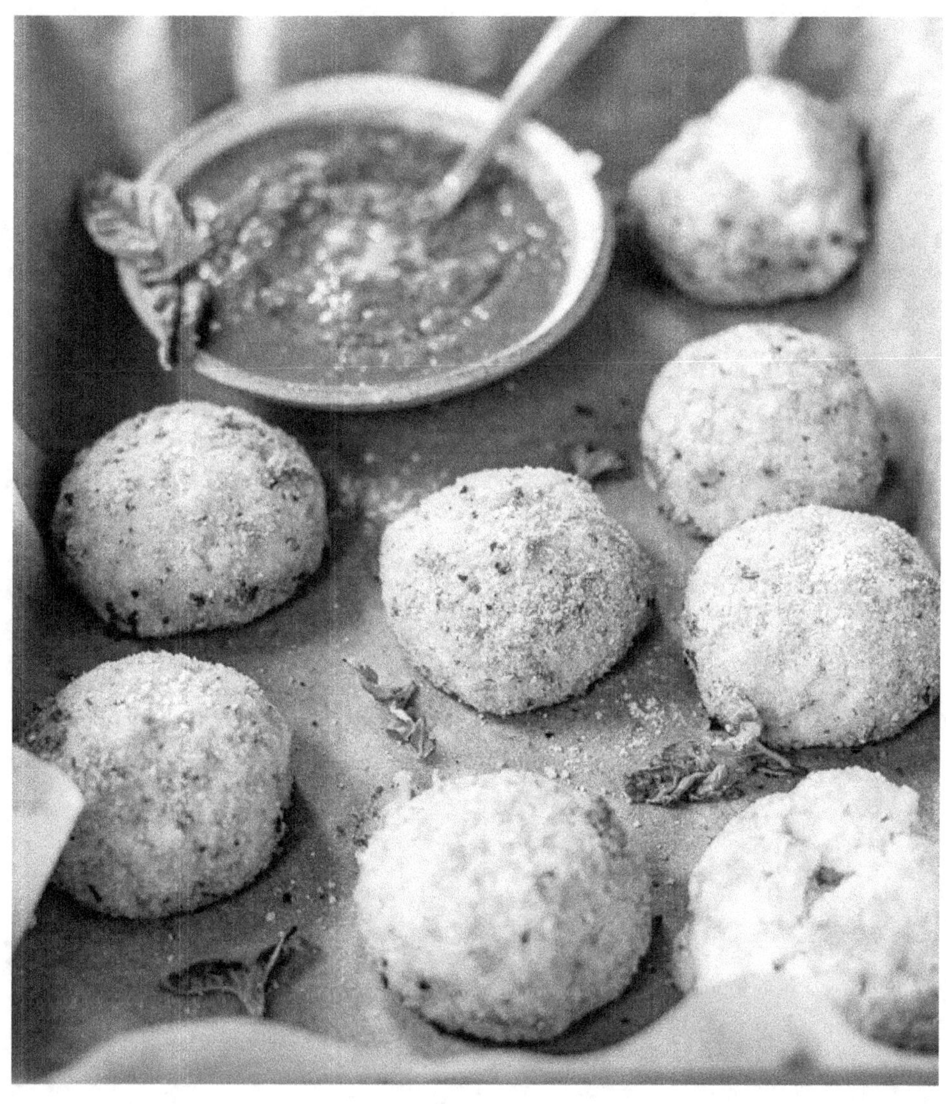

SMOOTHIES
&
BEVERAGES

40. RASPBERRY CHOCOLATE SHAKE

Ingredients

For 2 servings

- 2 cups unsweetened vanilla-flavored almond milk
- ½ cup sugar- free chocolate-flavored protein powder
- 1 cup fresh raspberries
- 2 tbsp coconut milk
- 2 tsp chia seeds
- 4 ice cubes

Directions

Total Time: approx. 5 minutes

1 In a large blender, process the raspberries, almond milk, chocolate-flavored protein powder, coconut milk, and chia seeds for 2 minutes until frosty.
2 Pour into glasses, place 2 ice cubes into each glass, and serve.

Per serving:

- Cal 219
- Fat 11 g
- Net Carbs 2.8g
- Protein 38g

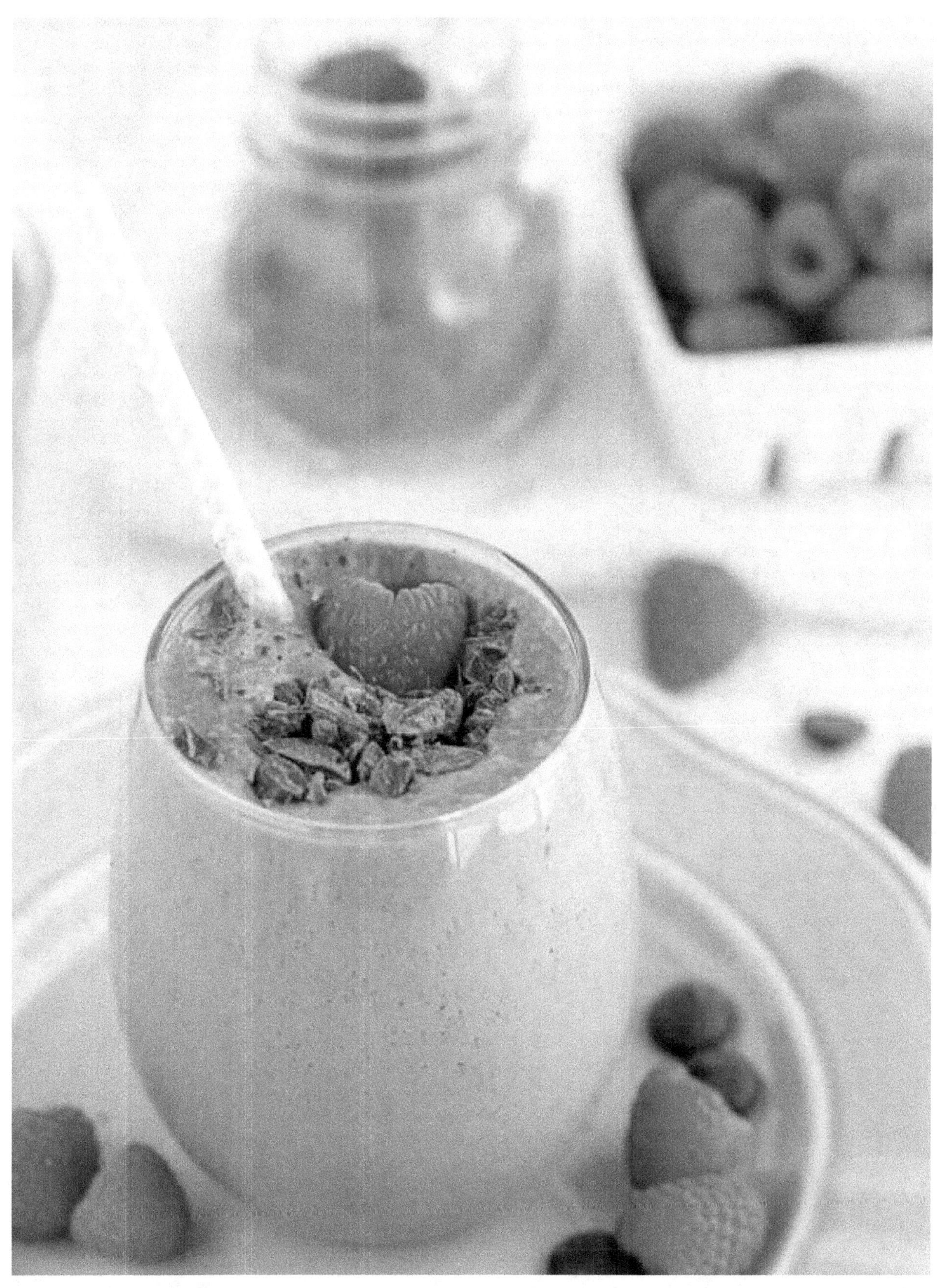

SWEETS & DESSERTS

41. CHOCOLATE CANDIES WITH BLUEBERRIES

Ingredients

For 4 servings

- 1 ½ cups blueberry preserves, sugar- free
- 10 oz unsweetened chocolate chips
- 2 cups raw cashew nuts
- 2 tbsp ground flax seeds
- 3 tbsp xylitol
- 3 tbsp olive oil

Directions

Total Time: approx. 10 min + cooling time

1 Grind the cashew nuts and flax seeds in a blender for 50 seconds until smoothly crushed; add the blueberries and 2 tbsp of xylitol. Process further for 1 minute until well combined. Form 1-inch balls of the mixture.

2 Line a baking sheet with parchment paper and place the balls on the baking sheet. Freeze for 1 hour or until firmed up. In your microwave, melt the chocolate chips, olive oil, and the remaining xylitol for 95 seconds. Toss the truffles to coat in the chocolate mixture, put on the baking sheet, and freeze up for at least 3 hours.

Per serving:

- Cal 253
- Fat 18g

- Net Carbs 4.1g
- Protein 10g

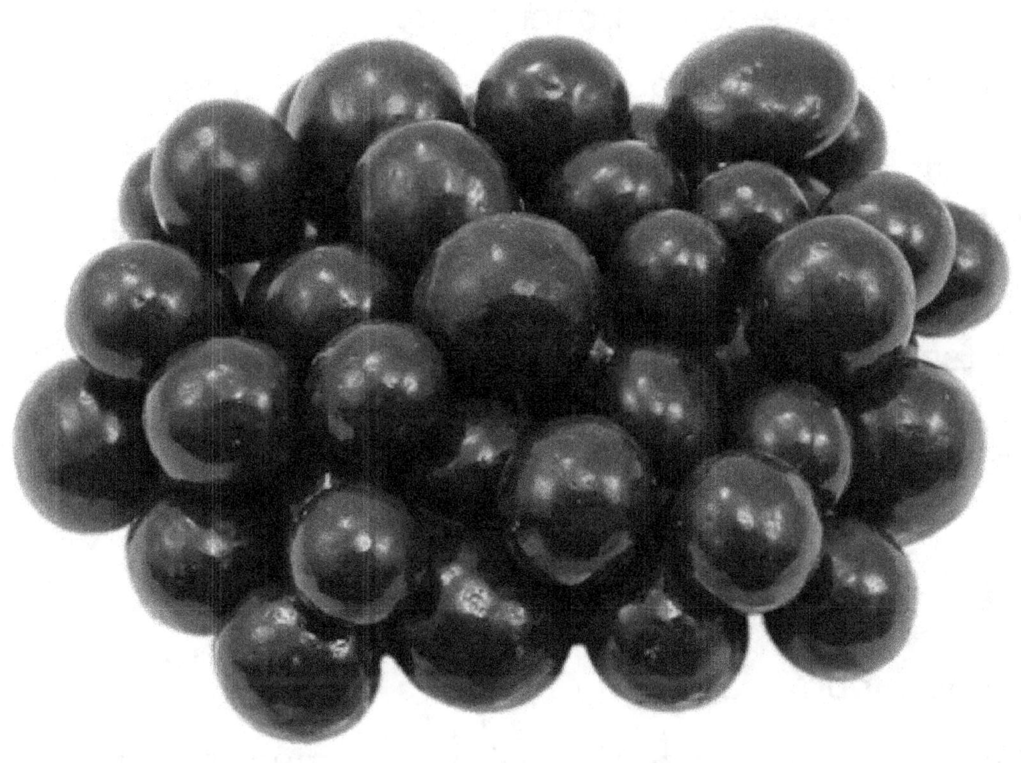

42. MATCHA BROWNIES WITH PISTACHIOS

Ingredients

For 4 servings

- 4 tbsp Swerve confectioner's sugar
- 1 tbsp tea matcha powder
- ¼ cup unsalted butter, melted
- A pinch of salt
- ¼ cup coconut flour
- ½ tsp baking powder
- 1 egg
- ½ cup chopped pistachios

Directions

Total Time: approx. 30 minutes

1 Line a square baking dish with parchment paper and preheat the oven to 350 F.

2 In a bowl, pour the melted butter, Swerve sugar, and salt and whisk to combine.

3 Crack the egg into the bowl.

4 Beat the mixture until the egg is incorporated.

5 Pour the coconut flour, matcha, and baking powder into a fine-mesh sieve and sift them into the egg bowl; stir.

6 Stir in the pistachios and pour the mixture into the baking dish to cook for 18 minutes.

7 Remove and slice into brownie cubes.

Per serving:

- Cal 243
- Fat 22g
- Net Carbs 4.3g
- Protein 7.2g

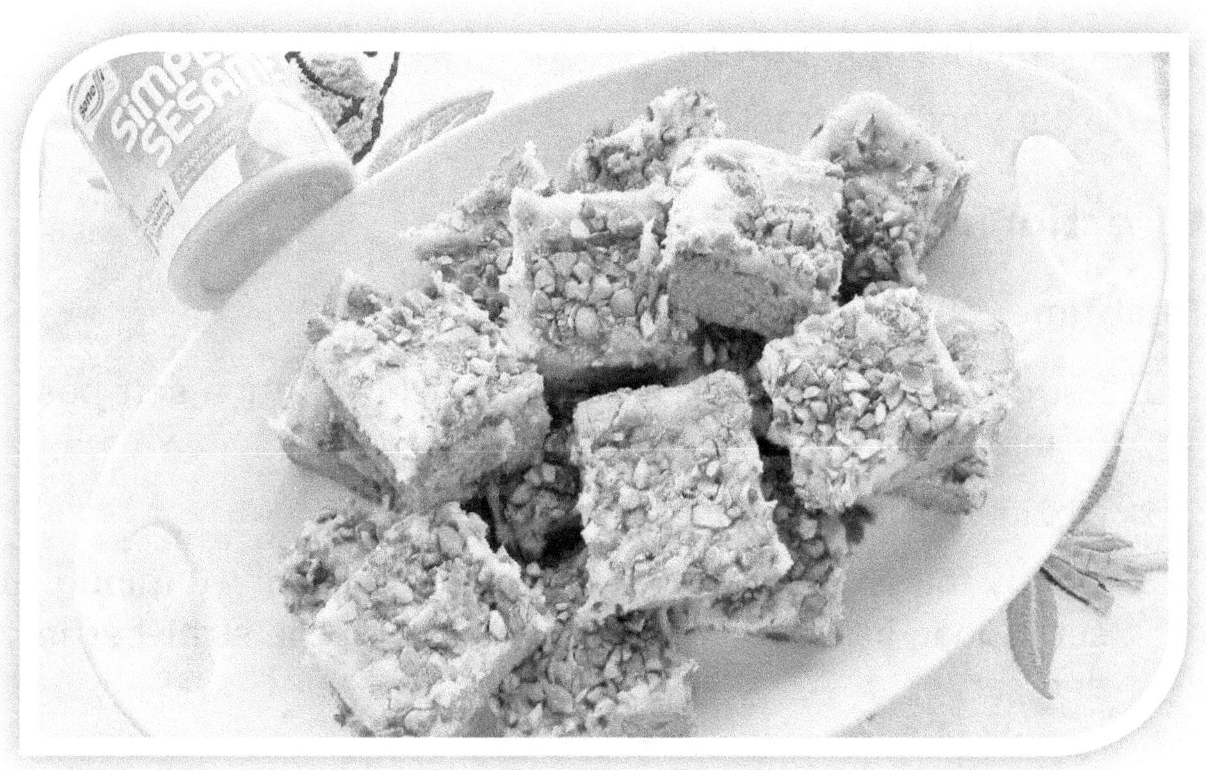

43. MASCARPONE & STRAWBERRY PUDDING

Ingredients

For 6 servings

- 1 cup mascarpone, softened
- 2 oz fresh strawberries
- 1 ¼ cups coconut cream
- 1 tsp cinnamon powder
- 1 tsp vanilla extract

Directions

Total Time: approx. 20 minutes

1 Put coconut cream into a bowl and whisk until a soft peak forms.

2 Mix in vanilla and cinnamon.

3 Lightly fold in mascarpone and refrigerate for 10 minutes to set. Spoon into serving glasses, top with the strawberries, and serve.

Per serving:

- Cal 231
- Fat 20g
- Net Carbs 3g
- Protein 6g

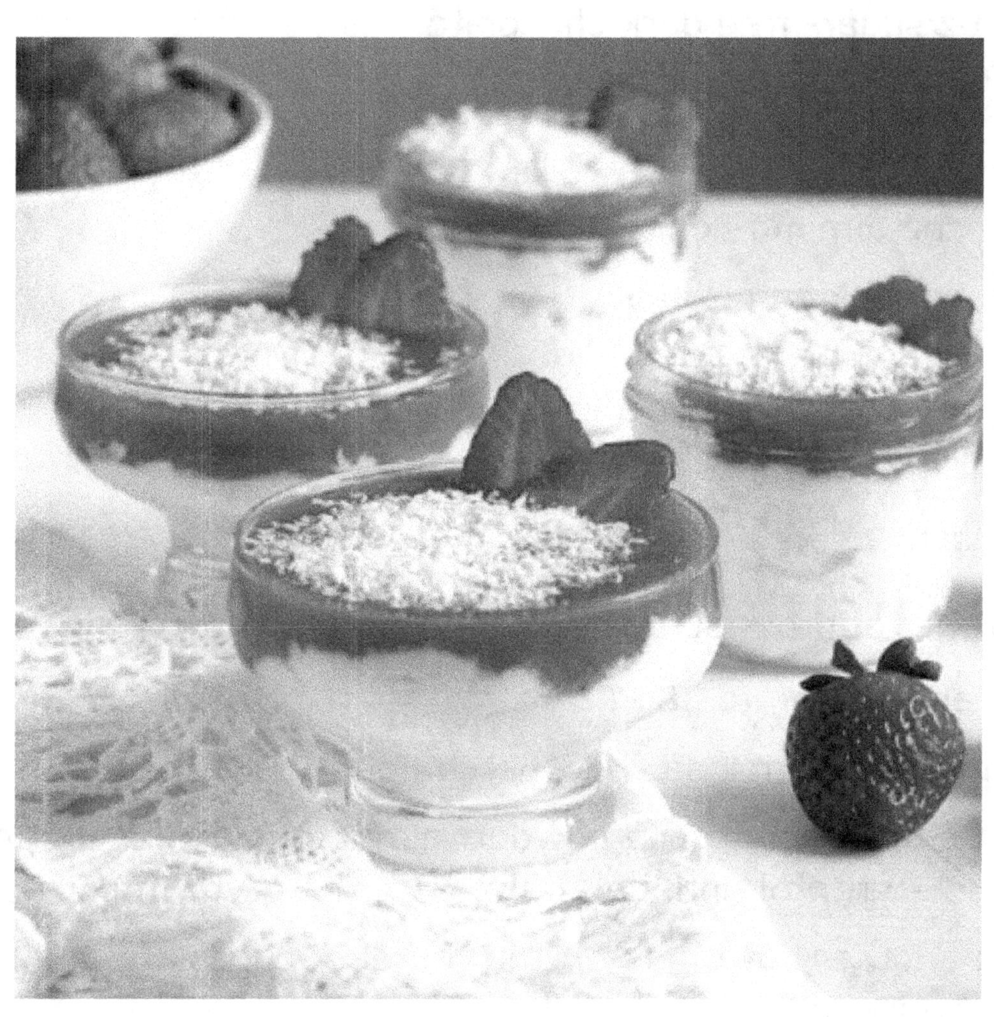

44. DARK CHOCOLATE BROWNIES

Ingredients

For 4 servings

- 10 tbsp butter
- 2 oz sugar- free dark chocolate
- 2 eggs, beaten
- ¼ cup cocoa powder
- ½ cup almond flour
- ½ tsp baking powder
- ½ cup erythritol
- ½ tsp vanilla extract

Directions

Total Time: approx. 30 min+ chilling time

1 Preheat oven to 380 F.

2 Line a baking sheet with parchment paper.

3 In a bowl, mix cocoa powder, almond flour, baking powder, and erythritol until no lumps from the erythritol remain.

4 In another bowl, add butter and dark chocolate and microwave for 30 seconds.

5 Mix the eggs and vanilla into the chocolate mixture, then pour the mixture into the dry ingredients; mix well.

6 Pour the batter onto the paper-lined sheet and bake for 20 minutes.

7 Let cool completely and refrigerate for 2 hours. Slice into squares.

Per serving:

- Cal 231
- Net Carbs 3g
- Fat 20g
- Protein 4g

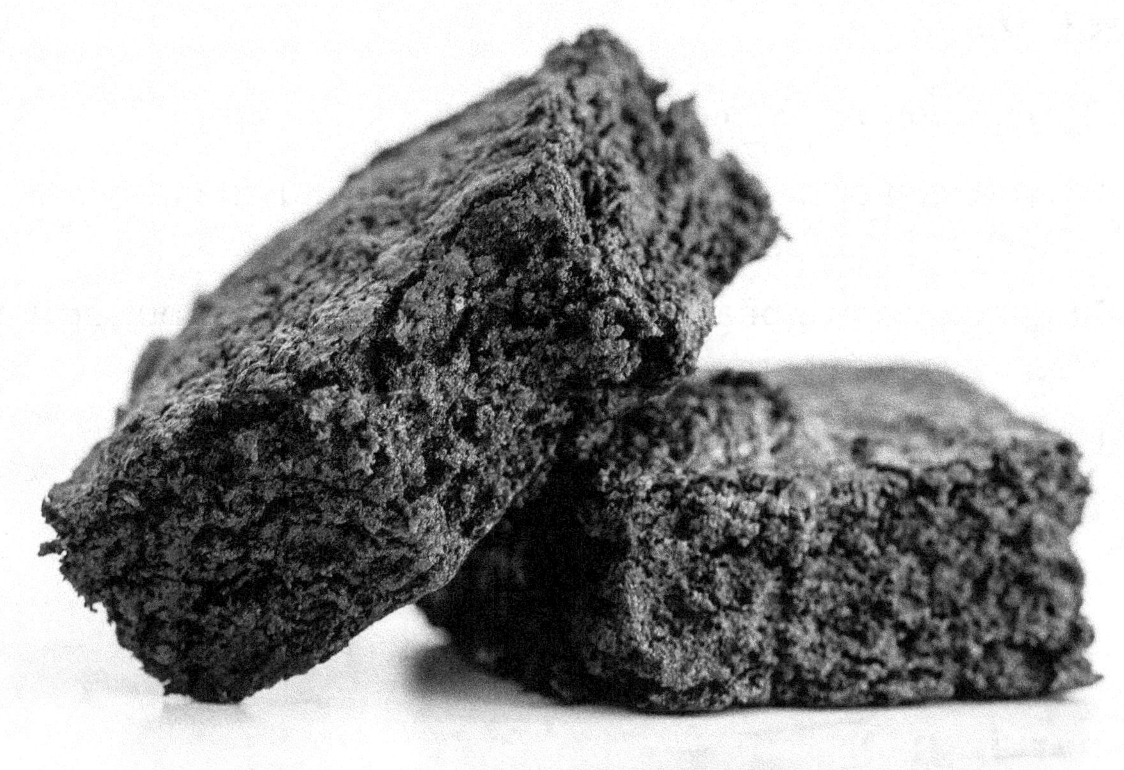

45. FAVORITE PEANUT BUTTER MOUSSE

Ingredients

For 4 servings

- ¼ cup smooth peanut butter
- 4 oz softened cream cheese
- ½ cup heavy cream
- ¼ cup xylitol
- ½ tsp vanilla extract

Directions

Total Time: approx. 15 minutes

1 Whip ½ cup of heavy cream in a bowl using an electric mixer until stiff peaks hole; set aside.

2 In another bowl, beat cream cheese and peanut butter until creamy and smooth.

3 Mix in xylitol and vanilla extract.

4 Gradually fold in the cream mixture until well combined.

5 If too thick, fold in 2 tbsp of the reserved heavy cream.

6 Spoon the mousse into dessert glasses and serve.

Per serving:

- Cal 229
- Net Carbs 5g
- Fat 21g
- Protein 6g

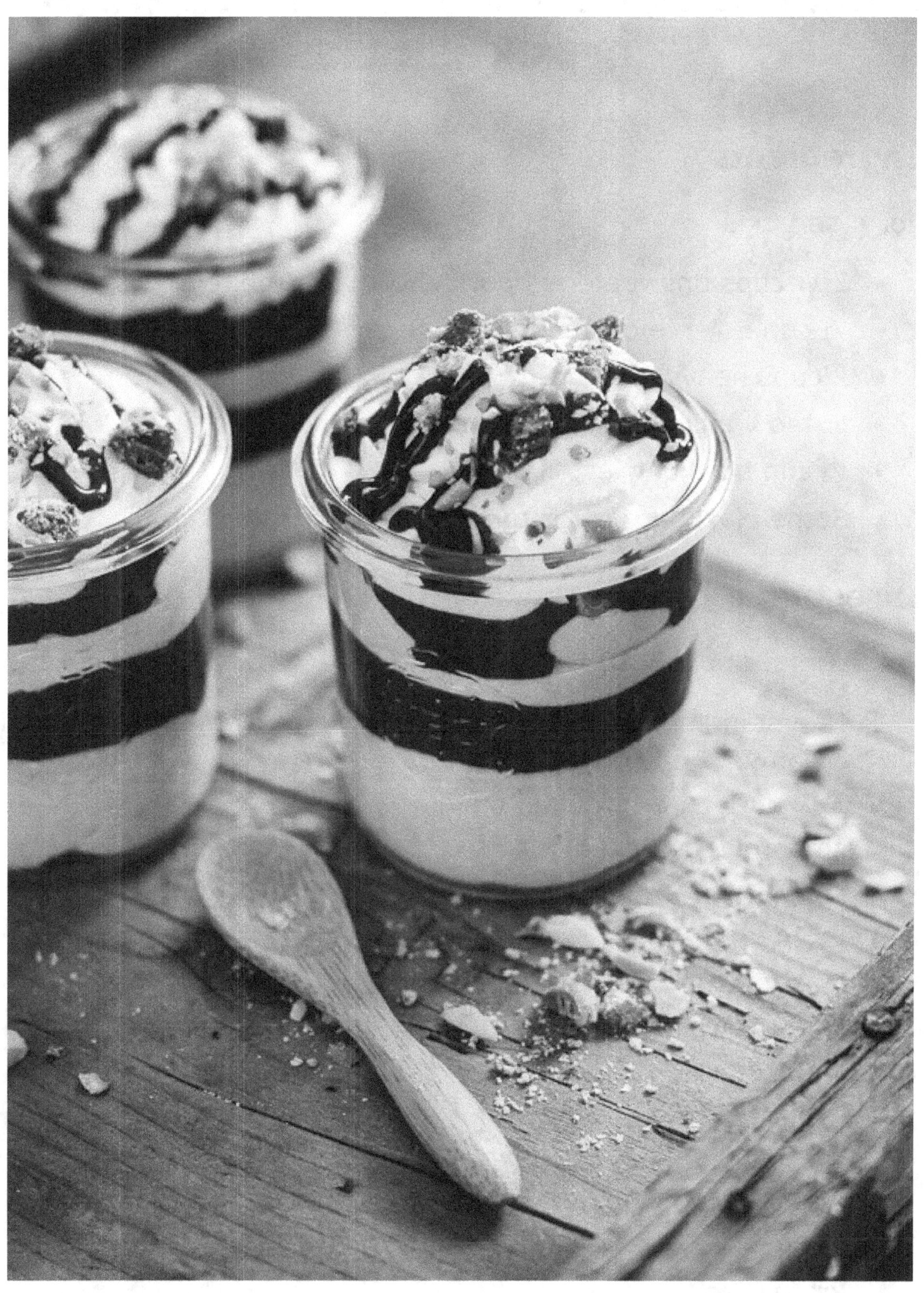

46. CHOCOLATE MOUSSE POTS WITH BLACKBERRIES

Ingredients

For 4 servings

- 2 ½ cups unsweetened dark chocolate, melted
- ½ cup Swerve confectioner's sugar
- 2 cups heavy cream
- ½ tsp vanilla extract
- ½ cup blackberries, chopped
- Some blackberries for topping

Directions

Total Time: approx. 10 min + chilling time

1. In a stand mixer, beat heavy cream and Swerve sugar until creamy.
2. Add dark chocolate and vanilla extract and mix until smoothly combined.
3. Fold in blackberries.
4. Divide the mixture between 4 dessert cups, cover with plastic wrap, and refrigerate for 2 hours.
5. Garnish with the reserved blackberries and serve.

Per serving:

- Cal 309
- Net Carbs 2.6g
- Fat 33g
- Protein 2g

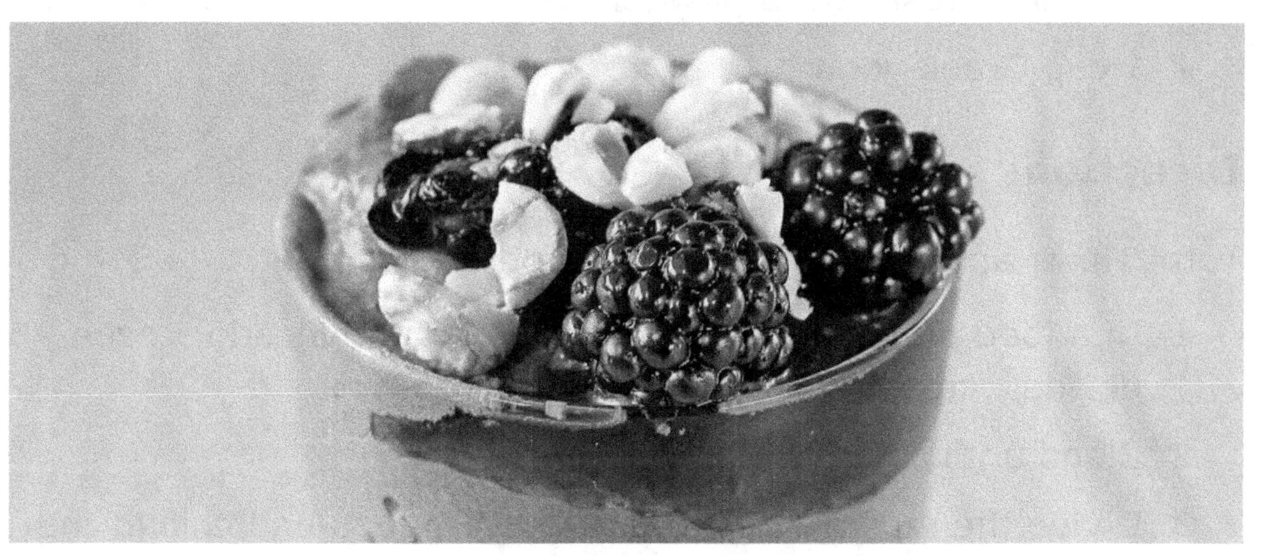

47. AVOCADO MOUSSE WITH CHOCOLATE

Ingredients

For 4 servings

- 1 avocado, pitted and peeled
- 2 tbsp cream of tartar
- 1 cup full-fat coconut cream
- 1 heaped tbsp cocoa powder
- 1 cup Greek yogurt

Directions

Total Time: approx. 10 min + chilling time

1 In a food processor, add coconut cream, avocado, cocoa powder, cream of tartar, and Greek yogurt.
2 Blend until smooth.
3 Divide the mixture between 4 dessert cups and chill in the refrigerator for at least 2 hours. Serve.

Per serving:

- Cal 329
- Net Carbs 8.2g
- Fat 31g
- Protein 6g

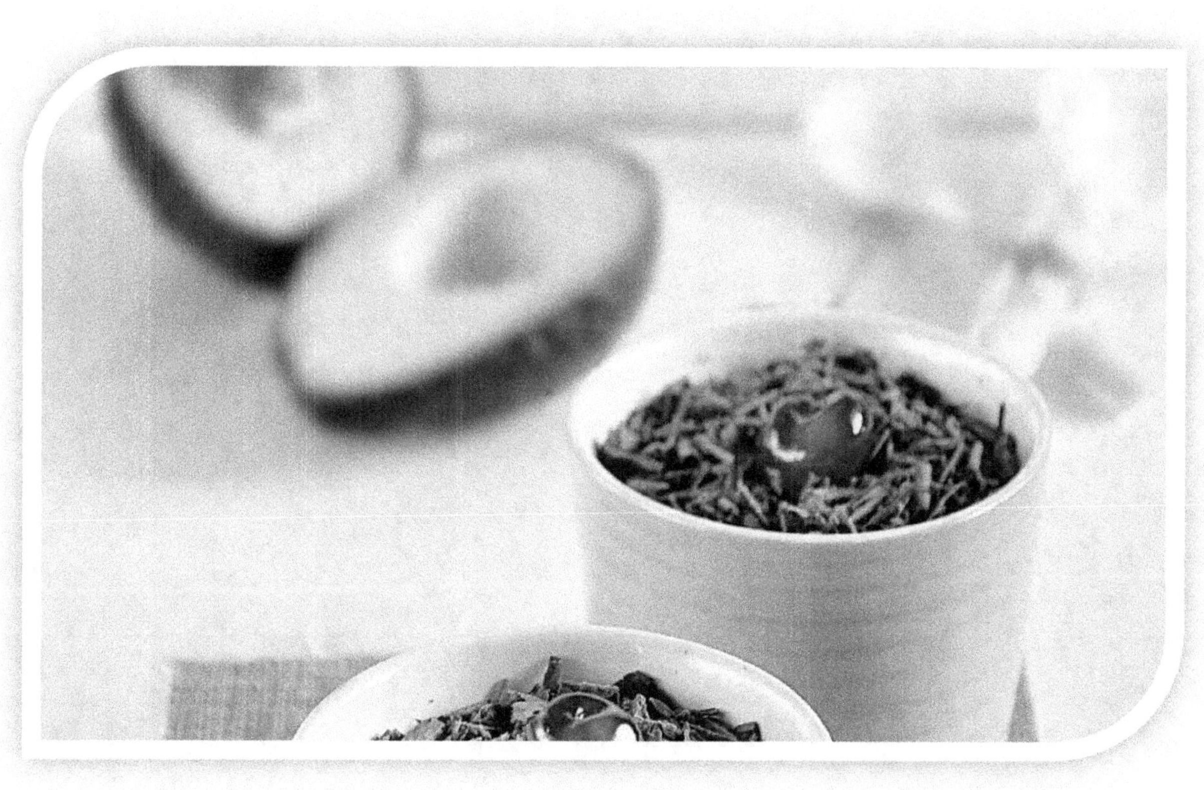

KETO SMALL APPLIANCE RECIPES

48. SLOW COOKER CHICKEN STEW WITH VEGGIES

Ingredients

- 2 garlic cloves, minced
- 1 cup mushrooms, chopped
- ¼ tsp celery seeds, ground
- 1 carrot, chopped
- 1 cup chicken stock
- 1 cup sour cream
- 1 cup leeks, chopped
- 1 pound chicken breasts
- 1 tsp dried thyme
- 2 tbsp fresh parsley, chopped
- Salt and black pepper, to taste
- 4 zucchinis, spiralized

Directions

Total Time: approx. 4 hours 15 minutes

1. Season the chicken with salt, black pepper, and thyme and place it into your slow cooker.
2. Stir in leeks, sour cream, celery seeds, garlic, carrot, mushrooms, and stock. Cook on High for 4 hours.
3. Heat a pot with salted water over medium heat and bring to a boil.
4. Stir in the zucchini pasta, cook for 1 minute, and drain.

5 Transfer to a plate, top with chicken mixture, and sprinkle
   with parsley to serve.

Per serving:

- Cal 312
- Fat 17g
- Net Carbs 8.4g
- Protein 26g

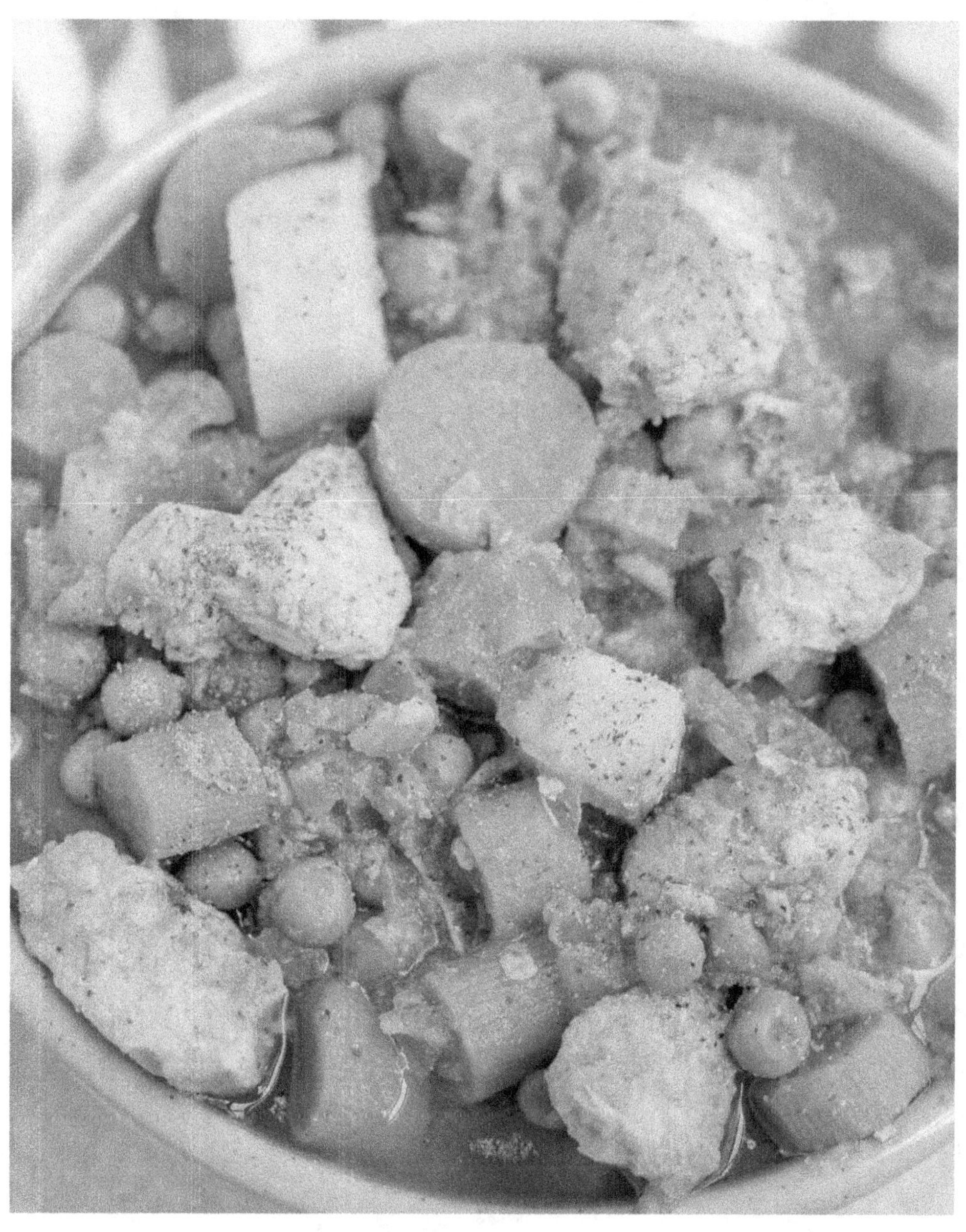

48. SLOW COOKER BEEF & BROCCOLI STEW

Ingredients

- 2 tbsp olive oil
- 1 lb ground beef
- ½ cup leeks, chopped
- 1 head broccoli, cut into florets
- Salt and black pepper, to taste
- 1 tsp yellow mustard
- 1 tsp Worcestershire sauce
- 2 tomatoes, chopped
- 8 oz tomato sauce
- 1 tbsp rosemary, chopped
- ½ tsp dried oregano

Directions

Total Time: approx. 4 hours 20 minutes

1 Coat the broccoli with black pepper and salt.

2 Set them into a bowl, drizzle over the olive oil, and toss to combine.

3 In a separate bowl, combine the beef with Worcestershire sauce, leeks, salt, mustard, and black pepper, and stir well.

4 Press on your slow cooker's bottom.

5 Scatter in the broccoli, add the tomatoes, oregano, and tomato sauce. Cook for 4 hours on High; covered.

6 Serve the casserole with scattered rosemary.

Per serving:

- Cal 677

- Fat 42g

- Net Carbs 8.3g

- Protein 63g

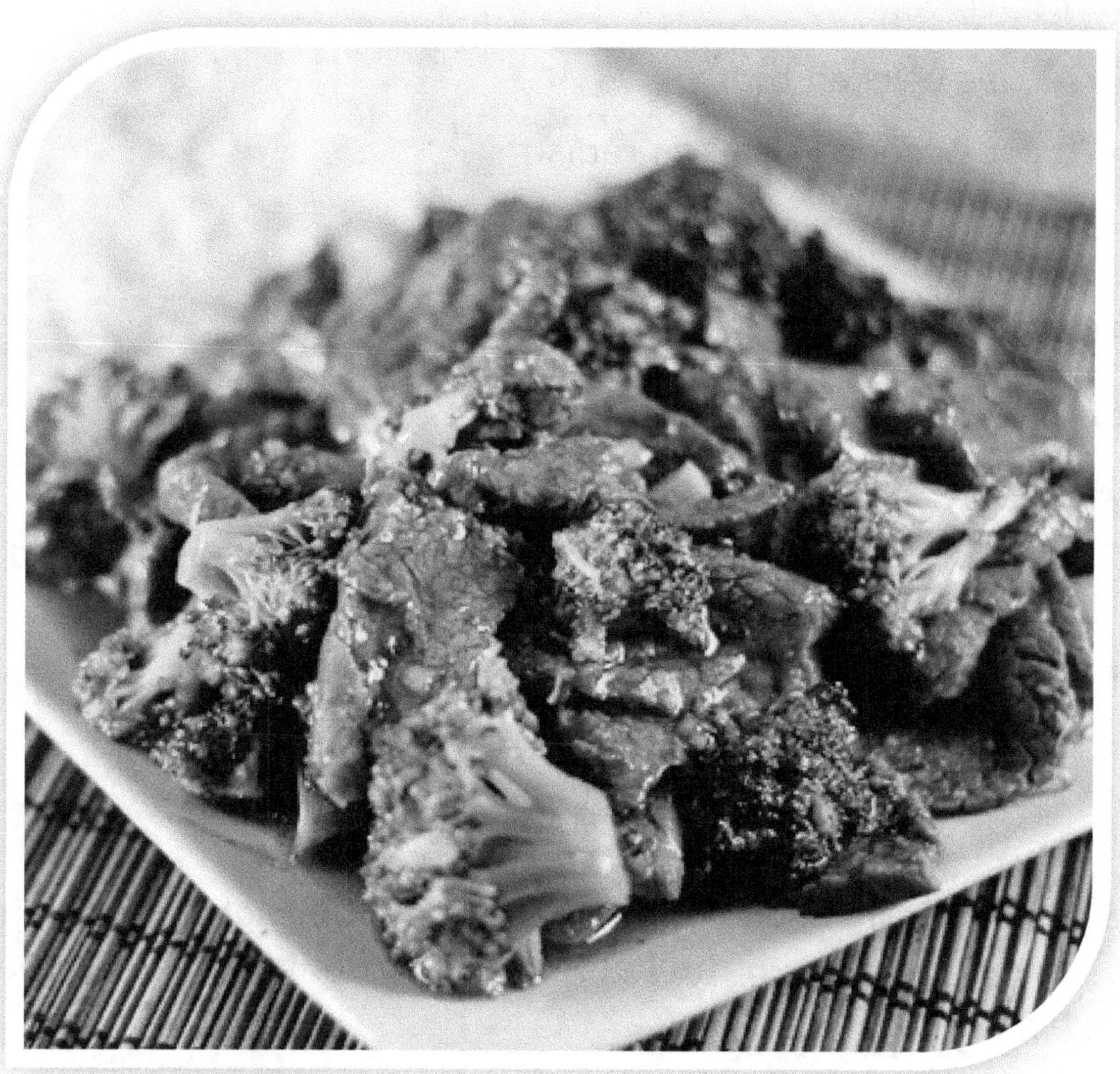

50. SLOW COOKER CHICKEN STEW WITH SORREL

Ingredients

For 6 servings

- 8 chicken breasts, cut into thin strips
- 2 tbsp olive oil
- 1 large leek, chopped
- 1 lb sorrel
- 4 cups chicken broth
- 2 cups chopped daikon radish
- Salt and pepper to taste

Directions

Total Time: approx. 4 hours 20 minutes

1 First, season the chicken with salt and pepper.

2 Warm the olive oil in a skillet over medium heat and add the chicken strips.

3 Brown the chicken strips for about 6 minutes; transfer to your slow cooker.

4 Top it with the leek, sorrel, daikon radish, and chicken broth.

5 Close the lid and cook the ingredients on High for 4 hours. Once ready, open the pot and adjust the taste with salt and pepper.

6   Spoon the stew into serving bowls and serve it with some
    cauliflower rice.

Per serving:

- Cal 260

- Fat 12g

- Net Carbs 2.3g

- Protein 22g

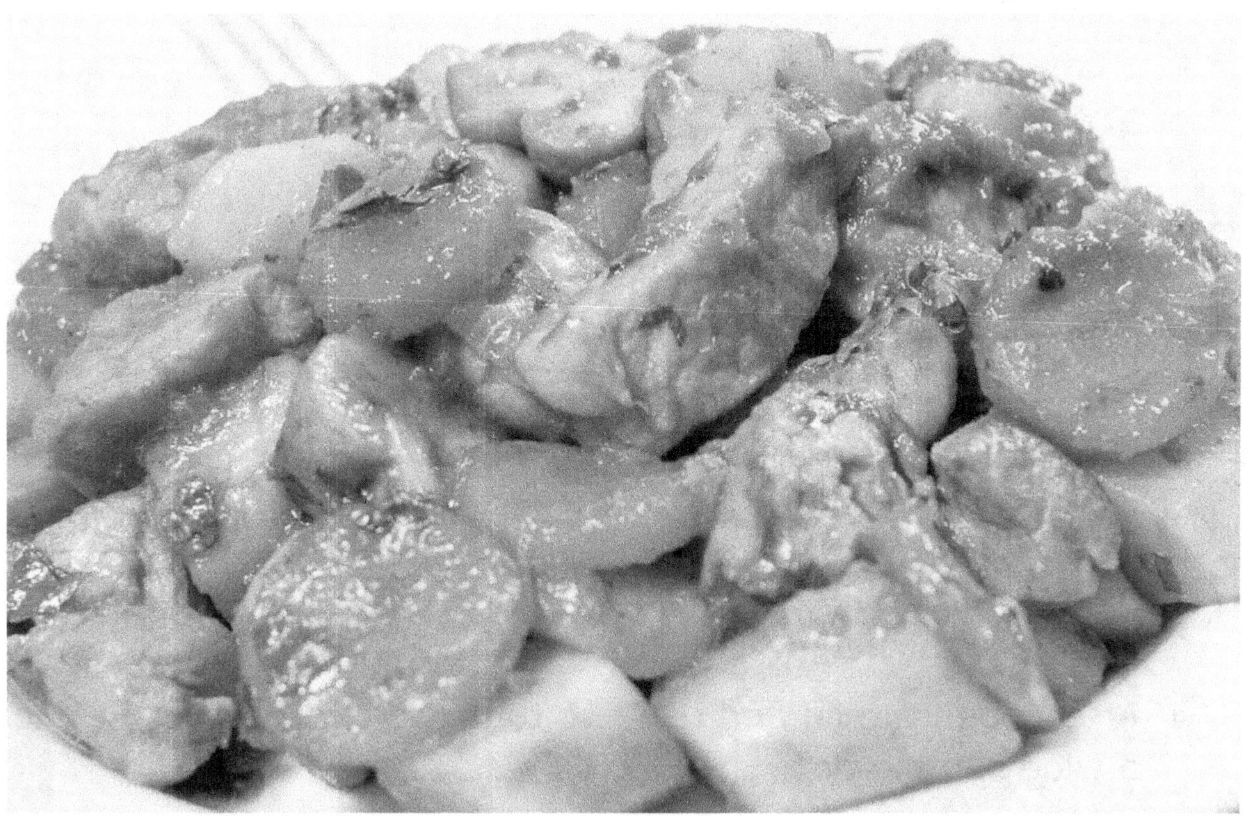

51. SLOW COOKER POULE AU POT

Ingredients

For 6 servings

- 1 (3.5-4 lb) whole chicken
- 1 brown onion, quartered
- 1 rutabaga, peeled and diced
- 1 celery stalk, chopped
- 2 carrots, diced
- 3 sprigs fresh thyme
- 1 bay leaf
- Salt and pepper to taste

Directions

Total Time: approx. 8 hours 20 minutes

1 Put the chicken in your slow cooker and place the rutabaga, carrots, celery, and onion around it.
2 Then, add the bay leaf, pepper, salt, and thyme and pour in 4 cups of water.
3 Cook the chicken on Low for 8 hours.
4 After, open the lid and use two tongs to lift the chicken into a wide serving dish.
5 Surround it with the vegetables and spoon some broth over them while discarding the bay leaf and thyme sprigs.
6 Serve and enjoy!

Per serving:

- Cal 210
- Fat 15g
- Net Carbs 3.6g
- Protein 28g

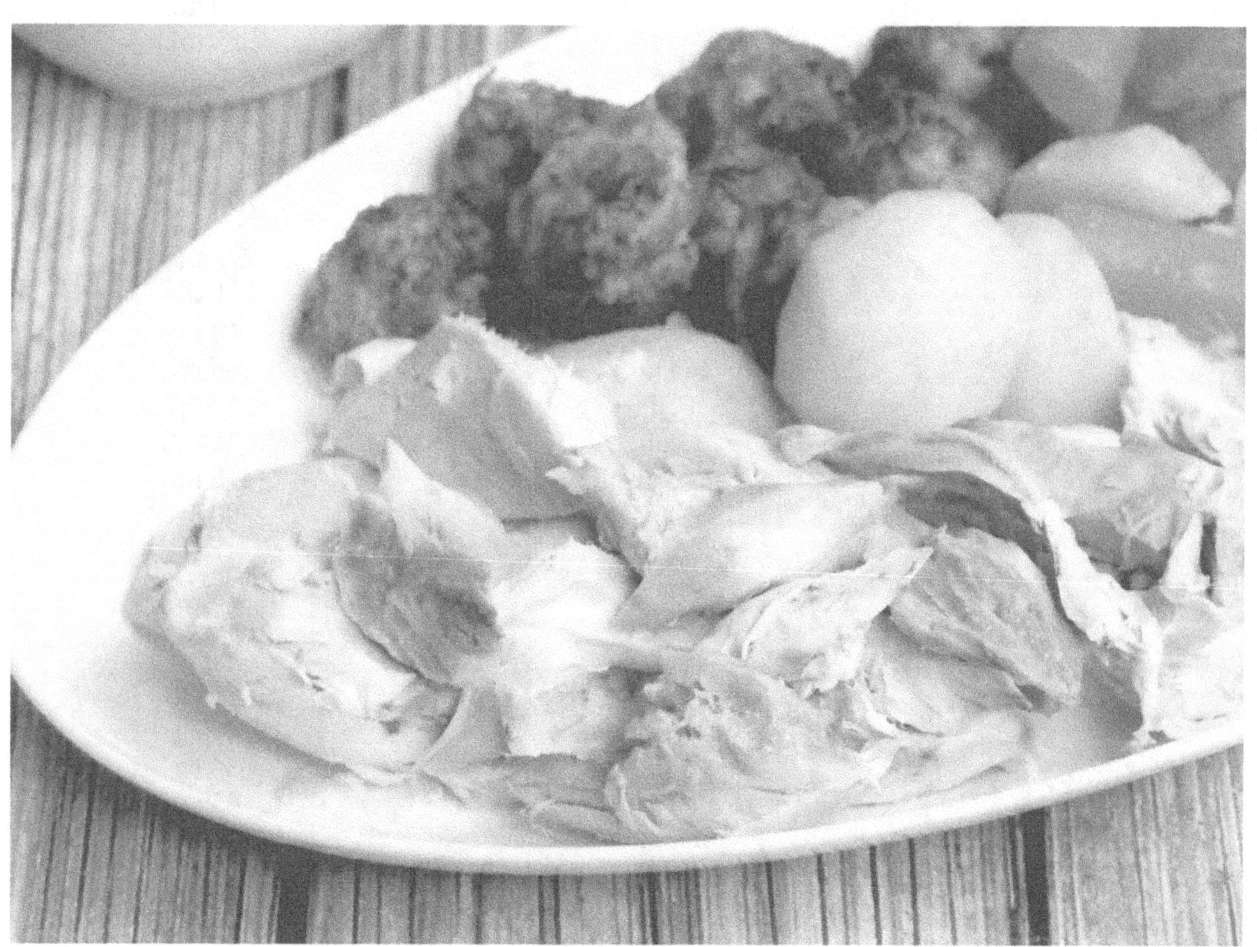

MEASUREMENTS & CONVERSIONS

	US STANDARD	US STANDARD (OUNCES)	METRIC (APPROXIMATE)
VOLUME EQUIVALENTS (LIQUID)	2 tablespoons	1 fl. oz.	30 mL
	¼ cup	2 fl. oz.	60 mL
	½ cup	4 fl. oz.	120 mL
	1 cup	8 fl. oz.	240 mL
	1 ½ cups	12 fl. oz.	355 mL
	2 cups or 1 pint	16 fl. oz.	475 mL
VOLUME EQUIVALENTS (DRY)	¼ teaspoon		1 mL
	½ teaspoon		2 mL
	1 teaspoon		5 mL
	1 tablespoon		15 mL
	¼ cup		59 mL
	⅓ cup		79 mL
	½ cup		118 mL
	⅔ cup		156 mL
	¾ cup		177 mL
	1 cup		235 mL
	2 cups or 1 pint		475 mL
	3 cups		700 mL
	4 cups or 1 quart		1 L
WEIGHT EQUIVALENTS	½ ounce		15 g
	1 ounce		30 g
	2 ounces		60 g
	4 ounces-		115 g
	8 ounces		225 g
	12 ounces		340 g
	16 ounces or 1 pound		455 g

	FAHRENHEIT (F)	CELSIUS (C) (APPROXIMATE)
OVEN TEMPERATURES	250°F	120°F
	300°F	150°F
	325°F	180°F
	375°F	190°F
	400°F	200°F
	425°F	220°F
	450°F	230°F